D1369780

DISCARD

Protecting
Data
Privacy
in Health
Services
Research

Committee on the Role of Institutional Review Boards in
Health Services Research Data Privacy Protection

Division of Health Care Services

INSTITUTE OF MEDICINE

NATIONAL ACADEMY PRESS
Washington, D.C.

NATIONAL ACADEMY PRESS • 2101 Constitution Avenue, N.W. • Washington, DC 20418

NOTICE: The project that is the subject of this report was approved by the Governing Board of the National Research Council, whose members are drawn from the councils of the National Academy of Sciences, the National Academy of Engineering, and the Institute of Medicine. The members of the committee responsible for the report were chosen for their special competences and with regard for appropriate balance.

Support for this study was provided by The Agency for Healthcare Research and Quality, and the Office of the Assistant Secretary for Planning and Evaluation, both of the Department of Health and Human Services (Contract No.282-99-0045, Task Order No.1).

International Standard Book No. 0-309-07187-9

Protecting Data Privacy in Health Services Research is available for sale from the National Academy Press, 2101 Constitution Avenue, N.W., Box 285, Washington, DC 20055; call (800) 624-6242 or (202) 334-3938 (in the Washington metropolitan area), or visit the NAP's on-line bookstore at **www.nap.edu.**

The full text of this report is available on line at **www.nap.edu.**

For more information about the Institute of Medicine, visit the IOM home page at **www.iom.edu.**

The serpent has been a symbol of long life, healing, and knowledge among almost all cultures and religions since the beginning of recorded history. The image adopted as a logo-type by the Institute of Medicine is based on a relief carving from ancient Greece, now held by the Staatliche Musseen in Berlin.

"Knowing is not enough; we must apply.
Willing is not enough; we must do."

—Goethe

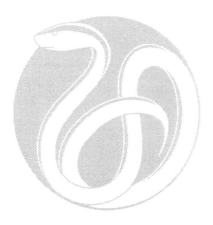

INSTITUTE OF MEDICINE

Shaping the Future for Health

THE NATIONAL ACADEMIES

National Academy of Sciences
National Academy of Engineering
Institute of Medicine
National Research Council

The **National Academy of Sciences** is a private, nonprofit, self-perpetuating society of distinguished scholars engaged in scientific and engineering research, dedicated to the furtherance of science and technology and to their use for the general welfare. Upon the authority of the charter granted to it by the Congress in 1863, the Academy has a mandate that requires it to advise the federal government on scientific and technical matters. Dr. Bruce M. Alberts is president of the National Academy of Sciences.

The **National Academy of Engineering** was established in 1964, under the charter of the National Academy of Sciences, as a parallel organization of outstanding engineers. It is autonomous in its administration and in the selection of its members, sharing with the National Academy of Sciences the responsibility for advising the federal government. The National Academy of Engineering also sponsors engineering programs aimed at meeting national needs, encourages education and research, and recognizes the superior achievements of engineers. Dr. William A. Wulf is president of the National Academy of Engineering.

The **Institute of Medicine** was established in 1970 by the National Academy of Sciences to secure the services of eminent members of appropriate professions in the examination of policy matters pertaining to the health of the public. The Institute acts under the responsibility given to the National Academy of Sciences by its congressional charter to be an adviser to the federal government and, upon its own initiative, to identify issues of medical care, research, and education. Dr. Kenneth I. Shine is president of the Institute of Medicine.

The **National Research Council** was organized by the National Academy of Sciences in 1916 to associate the broad community of science and technology with the Academy's purposes of furthering knowledge and advising the federal government. Functioning in accordance with general policies determined by the Academy, the Council has become the principal operating agency of both the National Academy of Sciences and the National Academy of Engineering in providing services to the government, the public, and the scientific and engineering communities. The Council is administered jointly by both Academies and the Institute of Medicine. Dr. Bruce M. Alberts and Dr. William A. Wulf are chairman and vice chairman, respectively, of the National Research Council.

COMMITTEE ON THE ROLE OF INSTITUTIONAL REVIEW BOARDS IN HEALTH SERVICES RESEARCH DATA PRIVACY PROTECTION

BERNARD LO (*Chair*), Professor of Medicine, Director of Programs in Medical Ethics University of California San Francisco

ELIZABETH ANDREWS, Director, World Wide Epidemiology, Glaxo Wellcome

JOHN COLMERS, Executive Director, Maryland Health Care Commission

GEORGE DUNCAN, Professor of Statistics, Heinz School of Public Policy and Management, Carnegie Mellon University

JANLORI GOLDMAN, Director, Health Privacy Project, Georgetown University, Institute for Health Care Research and Policy

CRAIG W. HENDRIX, Associate Professor of Medicine, Johns Hopkins University

MARK C. HORNBROOK, Associate Director, Center for Health Research, Kaiser Permanente Northwest

LISA IEZZONI, Professor of Medicine, Harvard Medical School, Beth Israel Deaconess Medical Center, Division of General Medicine and Primary Care

DONALD KORNFELD, Associate Dean Faculty of Medicine, Chairman, Institutional Review Board, Professor of Psychiatry, Columbia University College of Physicians and Surgeons, Presbyterian University

ELLIOT STONE, Executive Director and CEO, Massachusetts Health Data Consortium, Inc.

PETER SZOLOVITS, Professor, Massachusetts Institute of Technology, Department of Electrical Engineering and Computer Science

ADELE WALLER, Partner, Bell, Boyd & Lloyd, Chicago

Consultants

BARTHA-MARIA KNOPPERS, Professor, Faculty of Law, Senior Researcher, C.R.D.P., Legal Counsel, McMaster Gervais, University of Montreal

ROSS A. THOMPSON, Professor, Department of Psychology, University of Nebraska

Staff

LEE ZWANZIGER, Senior Program Officer
RITA GASKINS, Senior Project Assistant

Preface

Health services research (HSR) exemplifies some of the greatest hopes and greatest fears for collecting and analyzing computerized personal health information. Information routinely collected in the course of providing and paying for health care can be used by researchers to investigate the relative effectiveness of alternative clinical interventions, of alternative methods of organizing, delivering, and paying for health care, and of a variety of health care policies. Such research may improve the effectiveness and efficiency of health care. For example, HSR has identified significant variation in outcomes of care for a specific health problem according to the specialty of the clinician, type of insurance or reimbursement, and gender or ethnicity of the patient. At the same time, using personal health information for such research raises concerns about privacy (whether participants should provide the data) and confidentiality (how the data may be used later). Such concerns are intensified because of public concerns that confidentiality is being eroded for many types of computerized personal information, ranging from credit card purchases to addresses on drivers' licenses. Concerns about maintaining confidentiality of medical information are particularly important because patients disclose sensitive information to physicians that they may not tell close relatives and friends, such as information about their mental health, alcohol and substance abuse, and sexual practices. Confidentiality of medical information used in HSR is particularly important because information on many individuals may be analyzed by researchers without their knowledge or consent. The very power of HSR, to juxtapose patient-level data from a variety of sources on a large number of patients, also raises the largest concerns about confidentiality. It is often not feasible to obtain consent from every patient in a large population to be studied. Even if consent were possible to obtain, the requirement of consent would likely lead to bias and invalid findings, because those who opt out might differ systematically from those giving consent. Thus, for important HSR to proceed, it is important that the privacy and confidentiality of subjects be adequately protected.

IRBs play a key role in protecting the subjects of research. This IOM committee was charged with identifing current and best practices of IRBs that review HSR, both HSR that is subject to federal regulation and research that falls outside it. Within restrictions of the scope and time, the committee found a number of examples of IRBs that had put into place thoughtful, effective measures for reviewing HSR. There appears to be considerable variation in how IRBs deal with such difficult questions as how to distinguish HSR from such activities as quality improvement, how to determine whether a HSR project is exempt from IRB review, and how to determine whether informed consent can be waived for a HSR project. If IRBs adopted the best practices more widely, the quality of HSR could be improved, and the public could be more assured that privacy and confidentiality were being properly safeguarded in HSR.

Identifying best practices for protecting privacy and confidentiality in HSR is a promising approach that needs to be further developed. Identifying best practices is a quality improvement technique that builds on the achievements of HSR investigators and IRBs on the leading edge of their fields. It stimulates an explicit discussion of ethical concerns about HSR and potential solutions. Best practices give IRBs the flexibility to respond to the particular issues raised by different HSR projects; a technique that effectively safeguards confidentiality in one HSR project may be inappropriate in another. Finally, the approach of best practices not only helps to bring everyone up to a higher level, but also raises the best level higher as improved methods, such as informational technologies, develop and spread.

At the same time, the effectiveness of IRBs in reviewing HSR will depend on organizational factors. First, authors of GAO reports and in the popular press have noted that IRBs often do not have sufficient resources to carry out their charges. The committee found that IRBs will need additional resources and training to oversee HSR better, since HSR differs in important ways from clinical research involving new drugs or invasive medical interventions. Second, protecting the confidentiality of personal health information in HSR is easier if health care organizations effectively protect confidentiality of electronic personal health information, whether used for clinical or administrative purposes. Finally, the committee found that many IRBs play an important role in educating investigators about the protection of human subjects in HSR. In the long run, such educational programs will enhance the quality of HSR proposals submitted for IRB review.

I was privileged to work with a committee that was so thoughtful, committed, and embodied with good sense. We were grateful to the IRB chairs and administrators, health services researchers, and leaders of health care organizations who shared with us their wisdom, experience, and commitment protecting human subjects. The IOM staff was extremely helpful in keeping us on track on a tight schedule. Lee Zwanziger was excellent in pulling together information and ideas from many sources into a coherent, readable report.

Acknowledgments

The workshop speakers, listed in the appendix, all were very helpful and generous with their time in preparing, attending, and participating in the workshop. The committee very much appreciates the information and insight they provided both in the workshop and in comments and suggestions afterwards.

Many individuals assisted with helpful advice and suggestions throughout this project. The committee particularly thanks Paul Clayton of Intermountain Health Care, Nancy Donovan of the U.S. General Accounting Office, Gary Ellis and Tom Puglisi of the (former) OPRR, Molly Greene of UTHSCSA, Erica Heath of IRC, Steve Heinig of AAMC, Jon Merz of University of Pennsylvania, Eric Meslin and Margorie Speers of the National Biothics Advisory Commission, Andy Nelson of HealthPartners Research Foundation, Erica Rose of SmithKline Beecham, Joan Rachlin of PRIM&R, Patricia Scannell of Washington University in St. Louis, Ada Sue Selwitz of ARENA, Alvan Zarate of the National Center for Health Statistics, and many others.

The committee appreciates the support provided by the sponsors of the project, the Agency for Healthcare Research and Quality (AHRQ) and the office of the Assistant Secretary for Planning and Evaluation (ASPE), both of the Department of Health and Human Services. The individual representatives of the sponsoring agencies, Michael Fitzmaurice (AHRQ) and John Fanning (ASPE) were very helpful throughout the planning and execution of the workshop.

At the Institute of Medicine, the study director greatly appreciated the assistance of Sue Barron, Jennifer Cangco, Claudia Carl, Mike Edington, Rita Gaskins, Linda Kilroy, Janice Mehler, Jennifer Otten, Sally Stanfield, and Vanee Vines, among others. Florence Poillon helped in copy editing the report.

REVIEWERS

This report has been reviewed in draft form by individuals chosen for their diverse perspectives and technical expertise, in accordance with procedures approved by the National Research Council's Report Review Committee. The purpose of this independent review is to provide candid and critical comments that will assist the Institute of Medicine in making the published report as sound as possible and to ensure that the report meets institutional standards for objectivity, evidence, and responsiveness to the study charge. The review comments and the draft manuscript remain confidential to protect the integrity of the deliberative process.

Ruth S. Bulger, Ph.D., Former President, Henry Jackson Foundation for Advancement of Military Medicine
Donna Chen, M.D., Assistant Director and Research Scientist, Southeastern Rural Mental Health Research Center, University of Virginia Health System
Helen McGough, IRB Director, Human Subjects Division, University of Washington
Joan Porter, D.P.A., M.P.H., Office of Research Compliance and Assurance, Office of Veterans Affairs
Patricia Scannell, IRB Director, Human Studies Committee, Washington University

Although the reviewers listed above have provided many constructive comments and suggestions, they were not asked to endorse the conclusions or recommendations nor did they see the final draft of the report before its release. The review of this report was overseen by Hugh H. Tilson, M.D., Dr.P.H., Senior Advisor to the Dean, University of North Carolina School Public Health, also of Glaxo Wellcome Company, appointed by the Institute of Medicine, who was responsible for making certain that an independent examination of this report was carried out in accordance with institutional procedures and that all review comments were carefully considered. Responsibility for the final content of this report rests entirely with the authoring committee and the institution.

Contents

Protecting
Data
Privacy
in Health
Services
Research

Executive Summary

Our medical system is changing, with choices to be made by consumers, providers, insurers, purchasers, and policy makers at every level of government. The need for quality improvement and for cost saving are driving both individual choices and health system dynamics. However, no one at any level can make these choices wisely without research showing the pros and cons of alternatives in health services. This information comes from data on the outcomes that individuals or organizations experienced with a particular input—the selection of a health plan, drug, or health care delivery model. Yet these same data are information (often personally identifiable health information) about individuals. Most individuals value their privacy and, when they have chosen to share personal information with a health care provider, are then justifiably concerned about possible breaches in the confidential handling of that information. The health services research that we need to support informed choices depends on access to data, but at the same time, individual privacy and patient–health care provider confidentiality must be protected.

HEALTH SERVICES RESEARCH AND
QUALITY ASSURANCE OR IMPROVEMENT

Health services research (HSR) is the study of the effects of using different modes of organization, delivery and financing for health care services. More precisely, a recent Institute of Medicine (IOM) publication explained, "Health services research is a multidisciplinary field of inquiry, both basic and applied, that examines the use, costs, quality, accessibility, delivery, organization, fi-

1

nancing, and outcomes of health care services to increase knowledge and understanding of the structure, processes, and effects of health services for individuals and populations" (IOM, 1995). HSR includes studies of the effectiveness of health care interventions in real-world settings, as contrasted with studies of the efficacy[1] of interventions (e.g., new drugs) under controlled settings such as a clinical trial.

As an applied field of study, HSR is closely related to nonresearch investigations that are directed toward assessing and improving the quality of operations in healthcare organizations. Indeed, HSR and health care operations form two ends of a continuous spectrum. Some HSR projects are clear examples of research; applying scientific methods to test hypotheses and produce new, gener-

---

BOX 1 Who Is the Intended Audience of this Report?

This report is for all types of professionals and organizations that use or disclose data on health services. Although the Department of Health and Human Services is highlighted, the report should apply as well to other federal departments and agencies that are involved in human subjects research.

For organizations that have institutional review boards (IRBs) and whose research is subject to federal regulation:

• The practices and recommendations highlight some practices already in place in some IRBs and suggest additional support for IRB activities.

For organizations that use or disclose data but do not have an IRB or whose work is not subject to federal regulation:

• The practices and recommendations emphasize that the protection of human subjects from risks, including nonphysical risks from use of data, are of concern to anyone who uses or discloses data.

Although not all organizations have IRBs, all human subjects should be treated with the same high standards. The committee urges organizations that do not have IRBs to adopt practices of reviewing proposed investigations to assure that data confidentiality will be maintained. The committee likewise urges organizations that have, as well as those that do not have, IRBs to adopt system-wide confidentiality procedures and policies to protect nonresearch and research data.

---

[1]The term "efficacy" refers to how reliably an intervention brings about a given result under ideal, controlled conditions. The term "effectiveness" refers to how an intervention performs in the complex and variable context of real-world use and practice.

alizable knowledge. Other projects are certainly clear examples of internal exercises to assess the quality of the operations of the specific organization with no intention of producing generalizable knowledge. Many of these quality assessment or quality improvement (QA or QI) exercises are never intended to have any application beyond the specific unit within the organization that carries out the operation. In fact, many projects may start out as operations assessment and then become more like research, and many research projects involve doing very much what would be done in an internal operations assessment. As a result, for many projects, it is difficult to decide whether they are more like research, or more like QA or QI.

The benefits to society of HSR studies include increased understanding of the results of policy changes and other systemic effects of health care delivery systems. The major risks to subjects in HSR are not physical risks, such as unknown side effects of new drugs or invasive medical procedures, but psychosocial and financial risks resulting from improper disclosure of personally identifiable health information from the databases. That is, the potential for harm comes about through possible breaches of confidentiality in handling private and identifiable health information. Examples of the kinds of psychosocial or financial risks that may occur include potential denial of health insurance coverage, difficulty obtaining employment, embarrassment, loss of reputation, legal liability, or anxiety about what the recipient of an unauthorized disclosure of information might do with it.

The protection of privacy is a fundamental value in our culture. Research leading to improvements in the delivery and outcomes of health care, however, may be possible only with analysis of databases containing personally identifiable health information. Privacy can be protected by limiting access to data, or properly de-identifying the data, and by establishing other strong safeguards to ensure confidentiality. HSR can be only conducted if researchers have access to data, so it is important to concentrate on de-identification and other safeguards. We must protect both individual privacy and the societal benefits of research in order to achieve the appropriate balance. This report aims to highlight some practices that protect privacy while allowing research access to data.

PROTECTION OF HUMAN SUBJECTS

The involvement of living human beings in research as subjects is governed by federal regulations when the research is federally supported or otherwise subject to federal oversight. The body of federal regulations about human subjects protection is called the *Common Rule*, since it has been adopted "in common" by many federal departments and agencies that conduct, support, or regulate research with human subjects. Each department or agency has codified the Common Rule in its own specific regulations; this report mainly uses the regulations for the Department of Health and Human Services (DHHS) are located at title 45 CFR part 46, subpart A, for example.

The main mechanism for protecting research subjects and for assessing the balance of risks and benefits of research is the *institutional review board*, or IRB (specified in 45 CFR 46). An IRB is a standing committee composed of scientists, physicians, and others not directly involved with the proposal being reviewed (The IRB's membership and function are defined in the regulations to ensure that it has sufficient expertise and diversity to provide appropriate review. Diversity should include gender, race, culture, and profession. In addition to scientists, the IRB must include at least one person who is not otherwise connected with the institution and at least one non-scientist.). IRBs review proposals for research on humans to make sure that risks to subjects are minimized, that the potential benefits of the research outweigh the risks to subjects, and that the subjects will be respected as persons and not just used as research subjects. Under federal regulations, IRBs are required to ensure that subjects first be fully informed of the risks and benefits of the research and then have an opportunity to consent or decline to participate in the research unless the IRB decides that consent can be waived.

When an institution receives federal funds to conduct research involving human subjects, the institution must promise the government that it will operate an IRB according to federal research regulations for that research. Privately funded research that will be submitted to federal regulatory agencies, such as the Food and Drug Administration (FDA), must also be approved by an IRB that complies with federal regulations for the protection of human subjects. These regulations specify that in order to approve research, the IRB must be satisfied that among other requirements (45 CFR 46.111),

- risks to subjects are minimized and are reasonable in relation to anticipated benefits,
- selection of subjects is equitable,
- informed consent is obtained to the extent required, and
- provisions to protect the privacy of subjects and to maintain the confidentiality of data are adequate.

IRBs face complicated decisions when reviewing HSR and deciding whether such research is eligible for a waiver of informed consent. HSR protocols often have characteristics, such as the absence of any physical risk to subjects, that may make them eligible for a waiver of the informed consent requirement or even for exemption from IRB review. Because many HSR projects depend on secondary analysis of databases of records previously collected for another purpose, the investigator may not have the ability to contact the original subjects, and even if locating them is theoretically possible, the number of individuals in question may be far too large to make contacting them practicable. Indeed, many HSR projects could not be carried out if consent were required. In such situations, an IRB may grant the investigator a waiver of informed consent. Yet, when the IRB reviews HSR, it must make sure that confidentiality risks are not overlooked. Finally, private organizations do their own HSR or have programs such as quality improvement that use similar data and methods; this research may not be covered by the federal regulations and these organizations sometimes do not have IRBs.

The committee supports the review of all HSR proposals by knowledgeable individuals who are independent of the researchers. Although not all HSR is subject to federal regulations, the committee also concluded that the review of HSR ought to follow the principles of these regulations. Such a review body might be designated by any of several titles. The term "IRB" is defined in federal regulations and therefore has implications of the extension of federal oversight in a new area. The term "privacy board" has been used in a rule that, as this report was being written, had been proposed but not finalized, and it may mean different things to different people. Throughout the report the committee has used the term "IRB" to refer to formally chartered review bodies that are required to follow the Common Rule and other federal regulations. The term "IRB or other review board" is used to refer to bodies that review research but are not necessarily required to follow these federal regulations, although the committee urges them to follow voluntarily the ethical principles underlying the regulations.

GOOD PRACTICES

The objective of this project was to collect, to the extent possible, from workshop participants and other contributors, current best practices that IRBs and other review bodies employ to review research proposals and to ensure that privacy and confidentiality will be maintained within a balance between risk and benefit. Good IRB practices should apply the principles of ethical human subjects research and also be feasible for the type of research and the type of organization in question. That is to say, if we agree that we want to support HSR and obtain the societal benefits of research, then we must identify and implement practices that are feasible but that adequately protect the subjects. The committee hopes that the practices highlighted in the following chapters will facilitate HSR with appropriate and feasible mechanisms for the protection of human subjects, and will stimulate the development and dissemination of more advanced practices in the future.

In highlighting the empirical collection of practices, the committee recognized that good principles are already codified in the federal regulations on human subjects protection, but that no amount of codification can provide adequate direction for the day-to-day, study-by-study, work of an IRB. In short, regulations and guidelines are important to provide norms, but they must still be implemented with the judgment and practical experience of individuals closest to the situation. This is what the local IRB system is designed to do. The sense of the committee is that the local IRB system is strong and fully capable of reviewing HSR for privacy and confidentiality issues. Any IRB or other review body that reviews HSR will, however, have to understand the special problems of HSR and how to apply the principles embodied in the federal regulations. The aim of sharing best practices is to support review bodies by compiling the good ideas that have already been developed by IRBs and put into practice. One challenge of the future will be to find the best means of disseminating these good ideas.

PROJECT AND SCOPE

The IOM Committee on the Role of Institutional Review Boards in Health Services Research Data Privacy Protection was formed in December 1999 to gather data on the current and best practices of IRBs in protecting privacy (complete charge is given below). Two DHHS agencies, the Agency for Healthcare Research and Quality (AHRQ) and the Office of the Assistant Secretary for Planning and Evaluation (ASPE), sponsored the project.

To address these tasks, the IOM assembled a 12-member committee with expertise in medical ethics, HSR, IRB function, statistics, computer science, law, and database management. The committee met by telephone conference in January 2000. The committee and the IOM then convened a public workshop in March 2000. The committee invited testimony from IRB chairs and administrators, health services researchers, and other officers of academia, government, and private industry (see Appendix B). The workshop also featured presentations of the drafts of two commissioned papers, one addressing special considerations of HSR and confidentiality when the data pertain to minors (see Appendix C) and the other presenting an international comparison of health information privacy standards (see Appendix D). In addition to the workshop, the committee posted an invitation on a list serve and on the National Academies' website to IRBs to contribute information (see Appendix A). The committee collected further information informally by e-mail and telephone. Although the committee received just a few responses to the posted call for information, those received were very informative. The committee noted that all the providers of information, including respondents to the call for information, those who briefed the staff by telephone, and participants in the workshop, are a self-selected group of professionals committed to the IRB process. Information collection was thus not systematic and random, but particularly targeted. The committee deliberated by telephone and e-mail, and in closed meetings in April and May 2000, about the practices described to it. Finally, the committee has summarized in this report the practices it heard that seemed to be most effective. The committee addresses privacy and confidentiality pertaining to data used for HSR conducted through analyses of preexisting databases. There are many other aspects of the privacy of electronic medical records that were beyond the charge of the committee. The information in this report however—its findings and recommendations—applies as well both to data previously collected for another purpose and now being secondarily analyzed and to data derived in other ways. The committee chose to focus its work on studies involving analyses of data already collected for other purposes because such studies pose the most difficult ethical issues regarding HSR. Although HSR that utilizes surveys and interviews also raises ethical issues, the contact between researchers and subjects allows the subjects to learn about the research and decline to participate if they so choose. The committee recognized the strong connections between these related matters and the question of protecting data privacy in HSR using existing data. The committee therefore asks readers to bear in mind that such related matters were not in its charge and the committee did not address them.

The purpose of this project was to provide information and advice to the sponsors on the current and best practices of IRBs in protecting privacy in health services research. The charge to the committee was given in three parts as shown below.

1. To gather information on the current practices and principles followed by institutional review boards to safeguard the confidentiality of personally identifiable health information used for health services research purposes, in particular, to identify those IRB practices that are superior in protecting the privacy, confidentiality, and security of personally identifiable health information.

2. To gather information on the current practices and principles employed in privately funded health services research studies (that are generally not subject to IRB approval) to safeguard the confidentiality of personally identifiable health information, and to consider whether and how IRB best practices in this regard might be applied to such privately sponsored studies.

3. If appropriate, to recommend a set of best practices for safeguarding the confidentiality of personally identifiable health information that might be voluntarily applied to health services research projects by IRBs and private sponsors.

RECOMMENDATIONS

This section presents the committee's recommendations and findings based on the available information from IRBs working under federal regulations, discussed in more detail in Chapter 3, as well as recommendations from Chapter 4, on public and private health care companies that may not have IRBs or be subject to federal regulation. Chapter 5 suggests some directions for further work.

Best Practices for IRB Review of HSR Subject to Federal Regulations (Chapter 3)

Recommendation 3-1. Organizations should work with their IRBs to develop specific guidance and examples on how to interpret key terms in the federal regulations pertinent to the use in HSR of data previously collected for other purposes. Such terms include *generalizable knowledge, identifiable information, minimal risk,* and *privacy and confidentiality*. Organizations and their IRBs should then

BOX 2 Highlights of the Recommendations

Institutional review boards should:

• Help develop, and make accessible to investigators, materials including specific guidance and examples showing the implementation and interpretation of federal regulations, points to consider regarding protecting privacy and confidentiality in HSR, and review forms specifically designed for HSR (3-1 to 3-3).

• Educate themselves about the specific features and methods of HSR, and recruit or retain expertise (either on the committee or through consultants) on confidentiality and security in HSR involving analysis of data previously collected for other purposes, including the risks of identification of individuals and the physical security of data (recommendations 3-3 to 3-5).

• Adopt the best practices of IRBs working under federal regulations, and apply these practices to the review of HSR that is not subject to federal regulation (recommendations 4-2 and 5-7).

Health services researchers should:

• Have all HSR reviewed by an IRB or other review board with sufficient expertise in privacy or confidentiality protection, regardless of funding source or whether the institution is required to have all research conducted under federal regulation (4-1).

• Educate themselves to be aware of the best available techniques for confidentiality protection, including being careful to collect and retain only those fields that are truly needed (recommendations 3-5).

• Voluntarily adopt and/or support the use of best practices for the review of HSR by IRBs or data privacy boards (5-9).

Institutions funding, sponsoring or publishing research should:

• Promote education for members of the IRB or other review board regarding the special issues of research using health information previously collected for some other use and its impact on the protection of the privacy and confidentiality of human subjects (3-5).

• Have comprehensive policies, procedures, sanctions, and structures to protect health data confidentiality throughout the organization when personally identifiable health information is used for research or other purposes (4-3 and 4-4).

• Ensure adequate administrative support and funding for their IRBs or other review boards and incorporate improvement of IRB operations into overall institutional master strategic planning (5-1).

• Voluntarily adopt and/or support the use of best practices for the review of HSR by IRBs or other review boards (5-9).

• Have all HSR reviewed by an IRB or other review board regardless of funding source or whether the institutions hosting the research or providing the data have agreed to carry out all research under federal regulations (4-1).

BOX 2 *Continued*

The federal government Department Health and Human Services should:

• Provide more specific guidance to IRBs, clarifying the range of discretion that local IRBs have to interpret federal regulations and continue or expand educational efforts, along with private organizations committed to HSR such as the American Association of Medical Colleges, Association for Health Services Research (now the Academy for Health Services Research and Health Policy), American College of Epidemiology, International Society for Pharmacoepidemiology, Professional Responsibility in Medicine and Research, and Applied Research Ethics National Association (5-2).

• Continue and expand efforts to encourage holders of personally identifiable health information to make this information available to researchers as public use files after suitable application of techniques to minimize the risks of identifiability, and ensure that the data provided for HSR use are prepared in a manner that protects confidentiality adequately, including covering the cost of preparing government-held personally identifiable health information, so that confidentiality can be adequately protected in HSR (5-3 to 5-5).

• Consider supporting studies on the feasibility of developing procedures for facilitating linkage of separate data files containing sensitive data from different sources to create analytical files that are anonymized or for which the probability of identifying subjects is low, and on the extent to which IRBs assess nonphysical risks to human subjects (5-6 and 5-7).

• Consider other changes in policy and procedure including changing regulatory reference to "exempt" and "expedite" in the case of HSR to "administrative review" (5-8).

---

make such guidance and examples available to all investigators submitting proposals for review.

The committee found that several topics cause considerable worry to investigators and IRBs because federal regulations are open to varying interpretations, with divergent implications.

• The first of these topics is what activities are considered research and what criteria are used to operationalize the distinction between research and other activities. A key feature of the federal definition of research is whether the activity contributes to generalizable knowledge. In trying to distinguish research from activities such as quality improvement that use similar techniques to analyze personally identifiable health information in databases, however, both the federal regulations and the interpretations of these regulations by the Office of Human Research Protections (OHRP, formerly the Office for Protection from Research Risks, or OPRR) contain insufficient practical guidance for investigators and IRBs.

- A second important issue is what constitutes identifiable information as defined in the federal regulations. Should data be considered unidentifiable if linked to codes in such a way that the investigator would have great difficulty reestablishing the identity of subjects?
- A third issue is what constitutes minimal risk in HSR research and, in particular, what steps to protect confidentiality of data in HSR suffice to allow the project to be considered as minimal risk. The issues of identifiable information and minimal risk have important implications for whether a project may be exempt from IRB review or receive expedited review or whether informed consent of research participants may be waived. The committee felt that it would be desirable that all such research proposals receive some outside review.

On all of these issues, IRBs should communicate more directly with investigators and give examples more specific than the guidance currently available in federal regulations and clarifications by OHRP. Clearer guidance would make IRB review more efficient as well as enhance the protection of subjects by helping to ensure that HSR projects incorporate confidentiality protections that the reviewers find important.

> **Recommendation 3-2. IRBs should develop and disseminate principles, policies, and best practices for investigators regarding privacy and confidentiality issues in HSR that makes use of personal health data previously collected for other uses.**

Confidentiality in handling health information is important for its own sake and for the enhancement of public trust in research. The committee heard several innovative and feasible ways to facilitate the maintenance of confidentiality. The committee found, however, that the possible identifiability of data in HSR is a continuum, such that absolute guarantees of confidentiality are impossible.

Many techniques work together to increase the safety of confidential data, including protecting the data from unauthorized access by tracking who reviews the file, storing identifying information or codes separately from the rest of the data, and protecting the data from being physically lost, stolen, or surreptitiously copied.

> **Recommendation 3-3. IRBs should redesign applications and forms (paper and electronic) tailored to HSR that analyzes data originally collected for other purposes and then distribute them widely (e.g., post them on-line) to assist investigators in writing the human subjects sections of their HSR proposals and in preparing applications for IRB review. IRBs should be knowledgeable about the differences between HSR and clinical research, and any forms developed should reflect these differences.**

A checklist or logical series of questions lays out the criteria that the institution has adopted to determine, for example, what constitutes research. These instruments are useful in several ways: they call the attention of investigators to ethical issues arising in HSR, and they help investigators to think through systematically the specific issues regarding IRB review, patient consent, and protection confidentiality. Here, for example, is one approach to classifying a project along the HSR to QA–QI spectrum:

The following are characteristics of projects using HSR methods that are research, not QA or QI:

- It explores previously unknown phenomena.
- It collects information beyond that routinely collected for the patient care in question.
- It compares alternative treatments, interventions, or processes.
- It manipulates a current process.
- The results are expected to be published for general societal benefit.

Recommendation 3-4. IRBs should have expertise available (either on the committee or through consultants) to evaluate the risks to confidentiality and security in HSR involving data previously collected for some other purpose, including the risks of identification of individuals and the physical and electronic security of data.

Many of the techniques mentioned can be highly technical and are evolving rapidly. In order to confirm that confidentiality will be protected in a protocol, the reviewers will have to have access either to members or to consultants who can advise them on whether the proposal includes feasible technical measures to protect the data or whether the proposal has overlooked some potential confidentiality risks. This training should include cross-cultural issues related to definitions of privacy of personal, family and group information, depending on the specifics of how such cross-cultural questions arise in the local situation.

Recommendation 3-5. Institutions that carry out HSR and train health services researchers should require that trainees, investigators, and IRB members receive education, with updates as technology changes, regarding the protection of privacy and confidentiality when using data previously collected for another use.

Education is critical not only for IRB members, but also for researchers, technicians, and any other employees who may come into contact with personally identifiable health information. Better education about how to protect confidentiality and possible sources of risk will help investigators design better confidentiality protection for their proposed studies from the start. Better education of all employees who may come in contact with the data will help raise the level of understanding and alertness throughout the organization.

> **Recommendation 3-6. Health care or other organizations that disclose or use personally identifiable health information for any purpose including research or other activities using HSR methods should have comprehensive policies, procedures and other structures to protect the confidentiality of health information and should have in place appropriate strong and enforceable sanctions against breaches of health information confidentiality.**

Access to specific expertise and enhanced general education are important, but the committee also observed that the human element of the research enterprise necessarily includes human potential for error and even malfeasance. Therefore organizations should complement and support the proactive strategies of expertise and education for better confidentiality protection with deterrents to wrongdoing. Such sanctions should be graded according to the offense (e.g., whether the incident was a simple mistake or intentional violation) and should apply not only to researchers but to all employees of the organization.

Best Practices for Review of HSR Not Necessarily Subject to Federal Regulation (Chapter 4)

A good deal of health services research is carried out by organizations that do not receive federal funds for research and are not subject to federal regulations. These same organizations are dedicated to delivering health care services and products, so they also engage in quality assessment and quality improvement projects. These activities may involve very similar methods and uses of data, but they may not be classified as research.

The committee was impressed with the commitment to privacy and confidentiality that the representatives of several private companies presented at the workshop. Companies appear to be at different stages of developing internal privacy or confidentiality policies regarding HSR and should be encouraged to continue to develop these organizational policies and procedures.

> **Recommendation 4-1. Researchers should have all HSR reviewed by an IRB or other review board regardless of the source of support or whether the research is subject to pertinent federal regulations.**

> **Recommendation 4-2. IRBs and other boards that review HSR that is not subject to federal regulation should assess their practices in comparison with the best practices of IRBs working under pertinent federal regulations and, when the latter offer improvements, adopt them. Alternatively, when their own practices are superior though**

not subject to federal regulation, they should share them with IRBs applying the Common Rule.

IRBs offer a review of research projects by knowledgeable persons not directly associated with the project. This independent review protects subjects of research because independent reviewers may identify concerns and suggest ways to minimize risks that were not apparent to investigators. The committee heard several examples of protocols that were or could have been substantially improved with respect to confidentiality by relatively simple modifications, for example, omitting identifying data in the record, such as a Social Security number, that was not actually necessary for the research. Research subjects, who undergo risks for the benefit of science and society as a whole, should have the protections of such independent review as a matter of ethical best practice, regardless of funding source. There is little ethical justification for making a distinction between the level of protection afforded subjects in federally funded projects and that given subjects in projects funded by private sources if the risks to these subjects are comparable.

As in Recommendation 3-2, IRBs or other review bodies should develop lists of points to consider on protecting privacy and confidentiality in HSR for use by investigators. As noted in Recommendation 3-3, the committee suggests that the development and on-line posting of applications and review forms specifically designed for HSR would improve the quality of review of HSR projects. IRBs and other review bodies in any setting should inform themselves about the differences between HSR and clinical research, and any forms developed should reflect these differences. As mentioned in Recommendation 3-4, IRBs or similar review bodies should have available expertise (either on the committee or through consultants) to evaluate the risks to confidentiality and security in HSR, including the risks of identification of individuals and the physical security of data. Also, as stated in Recommendation 3-5, organizations should require that researchers and other employees who come in contact with confidential health information receive education in the handling of this information to maintain confidentiality.

Recommendation 4-3. Health care organizations that conduct projects applying the methods of HSR to personally identifiable health information for purposes such as QA or QI, disease management, and core business functions as well as for research should have comprehensive policies, procedures, and other structures to protect health privacy when personally identifiable health information is used for research or other purposes.

Recommendation 4-4. Health care or other organizations that disclose or use personally identifiable health information for any purpose including QA or QI, disease management, and core business functions as well as for research should have in place appropriate,

strong, and enforceable sanctions against breaches of the confidentiality of health information.

The members of the committee agreed that previous experience provides ample evidence that, although most investigators and staff are upstanding, there will always be a few who are subject to the temptation to misuse access to confidential information or who maintain records in an insecure manner. In fact, the committee felt that this aspect of human subjects protection may have been neglected and therefore recommends consideration of deterrent policies both for organizations working with IRBs under the Common Rule and for those that do not.

Large health care organizations reported that most violations of confidentiality occurred outside the research arena, in such areas as clinical care and business activities. This distribution is not surprising because most uses of personally identifiable health information are in these nonresearch areas. From the viewpoint of the patient, it does not matter whether a violation of confidentiality occurs in a research project or other activity because the risks of being harmed or wronged may be the same.

Recommendations for Next Steps (Chapter 5)

"The end of this study will not be the end of studying [the issue of privacy and confidentiality in health services research]," said Dr. Michael Fitzmaurice of AHRQ, one of the sponsoring agencies, during the committee's workshop. The committee appreciated that the charge of this particular study was focused and accordingly endeavored to stay strictly within the charge. In the course of the study, however, the committee found many important questions that would seem to be answerable in practical terms, although doing so would be far beyond the scope of this report. The present project has, however, brought these other issues into a new sharper focus. The committee's suggestions for further work and future steps may communicate this vision to others.

Recommendation 5-1. Institutions whose IRBs or other review boards review HSR should ensure adequate administrative support and funding for review bodies and should incorporate improving review operations into overall institutional strategic planning, and organizations that sponsor HSR should also support designating adequate funds for such review.

The committee corroborated previous reports that questioned whether IRBs have the resources to carry out their mission. The committee noted especially the April 2000 update report of the DHHS Office of the Inspector General (OIG). This report, *Protecting Human Research Subjects: Status of Recommendations*, concluded that the resource problems identified in the OIG's 1998 report, *Institutional Review Boards: A Time for Reform*, still exist. The committee heard that many IRBs already have a heavy workload of proposals for review, and that most members serve in a voluntary capacity. In addition, the practices that the committee heard and believes can be positive facilitators of IRB quality and efficiency in the review of HSR will require investment on the part of the IRB's institutional home in computer equipment, applications development, and expertise to support these programs and advise the organization.

> **Recommendation 5-2. The DHHS and other federal departments and private organizations such as the Association of American Medical Colleges, the Association for Health Services Research (now the Academy for Health Services Research and Health Policy), the American College of Epidemiology, the International Society for Pharmacoepidemiology, Public Responsibility in Medicine and Research, the Applied Research Ethics National Association, and others should continue or expand educational efforts regarding the protection of the confidentiality of personally identifiable health information in research.**

While these recommendations highlight DHHS as the sponsor of this study and a major sponsor of relevant research, the recommendations should be applied by other Common Rule signatory departments and agencies as well. The committee believes that the approach of identifying best practices for IRB oversight of HSR is a fruitful one that should to be further developed. Recommendations of best practices will provide more specific guidance to investigators and IRB members than is currently available, and IRBs will continue to devise additional good practices. This approach draws its strength from the commitment both of IRB members and administrators and of researchers to protecting the rights and welfare of the subjects of HSR. Both IRBs and scientists have developed useful practices that, if more widely adopted, could lead to improved protection of confidentiality and privacy, without creating undue burdens.

> **Recommendation 5-3. Organizations that furnish health services researchers with personally identifiable health information should ensure that the data are prepared in a manner that protects confidentiality adequately.**

The committee heard several instances reported at the workshop where HSR investigators requested de-identified data from federal agencies but received data that had not been de-identified because the agency in question lacked the resources to do so.

As large holders of personally identifiable data, federal agencies should not be in the situation of having to choose between providing data that have not been de-identified, or simply refusing to provide data for research at all. Organizations holding personally identifiable health data should develop and/or implement lists of points to consider in reviewing data requests with respect to protecting privacy and confidentiality in HSR.

Recommendation 5-4. The funders of HSR should be willing to cover the cost of preparing personally identifiable health information that is collected in clinical care, billing, or payment so that confidentiality can be adequately protected in HSR.

Recommendation 5-5. The DHHS should continue and expand efforts to encourage holders of personally identifiable health information to make this information available to researchers as public use files after suitable application of techniques to minimize the risks of identifiability.

If an organization holding health data has made a dataset publicly available without restriction, as is done with the National Health Interview Survey (NHIS), then projects using only such data can be considered minimal risk and eligible for exemption per 45 CFR 46.101(b)(5). In order to promote HSR, data-holding organizations should consider making as much data available in the public domain as is safely possible. The committee notes that the Interagency Confidentiality and Data Access Group (affiliated with the Federal Committee on Statistical Methodology) has developed a checklist for use in considering whether data may be released, which helps holders of data develop such public use files.[2]

Recommendation 5-6. The AHRQ should consider supporting a feasibility study on developing procedures for facilitating linkage of separate data files containing sensitive data from different sources to create analytical files such that it would be possible for researchers to create linkages that are reliable and informative, and at the same time, to protect the confidentiality of the original data disclosure through de-identification and other protective measures so as to save the subject from being placed at risk of harm or wrong through improper re-identification.

Much of the value of retrospective, database-oriented research comes from the ability to draw inferences from data derived from different sources. The committee urges interested parties, including DHHS agencies, to encourage research on linkage and anonymization with a view toward two goals: first, it should be possible for researchers to create linkages that are reliable and informative, and second, we should approach as closely as possible the goal of

---

[2]Confidentiality and Data Access Committee, Federal Committee on Statistical Methodology. Checklist on Disclosure Potential of Proposed Data Releases (July 1999): http://www.fcsm.gov/spwptbco.html.

anonymized data. Ideally then, the various sources of data would have their records indexed by the same set of identifiers, but ones that are not easily reassociated with the actual patient's identity. There are several possible ways to address this problem. One suggestion exploits developing cryptographic and authentication technology to create flexible health information identification systems (as explored in a pilot study of Kohane et al., 1998). Another type of linkage system would depend on trusted third parties with no interest in either data collection or the research project to be responsible for linking the separate data files. These entities could hold the keys linking individuals to the data. After merging datasets, this entity would then strip off the identifiers, check that identification cannot be (reasonably) inferred,[3] and take any needed steps to protect the data. There are positive and negative aspects to either approach, so the feasibility of both should be further tested.

Recommendation 5-7. DHHS (AHRQ and/or the NIH) should consider developing and supporting a research agenda concerning IRB protection of subjects from nonphysical harms such as risks to privacy and confidentiality in human subjects research (including cultural meanings of privacy and confidentiality).

A systematic study of nonphysical risk assessment was beyond the charge given to this IOM committee, and the committee would in any case have found itself unable to accomplish it due to time limitations and rules of the Office of Management and Budget requiring additional clearance for extensive surveys. The committee found, however, that such information would be of great use both as a baseline and, if updated periodically, as a basis of continuous policy evaluation. Such a research agenda would likely include current IRB practice as well as new procedures and policies to provide better human subjects protection and also would include monitoring of IRB practices. The findings would be of use to IRBs, researchers, regulators, and any other parties interested in privacy and confidentiality.

Recommendation 5-8. The OHRP should review the possibility of proposing a change to the regulations with respect to HSR to replace the terms "exempt" and "expedite" with "administrative review."

The committee is recommending this only with respect to HSR, not having investigated possible consequences for other types of research. The committee heard several reports that well-intentioned and conscientious researchers may judge a study to be exempt from review under the current regulatory language and therefore never bring it to the attention of a review board. Since the com-

---

[3]The committee recognizes that the question of how difficult identifiability by inference must be in order to make data safe for release will continue to be a matter of debate and notes that the standard should be expected to change as technology changes.

mittee has concluded that all HSR should receive some review by a board that is independent of the research project, the committee suggests that this possibly misleading terminology be avoided. The committee recognizes, however, that a change to the Common Rule involves coordination among many agencies. The committee further recognizes that others may have other suggestions for a new term. The committee's goal in this matter was to offer a term that recognized that some studies do not need full IRB review but does not seem to suggest that the investigator should decide what level of IRB review is needed.

Recommendation 5-9. Health services researchers, and institutions that participate in and benefit from HSR, should voluntarily adopt best practices for IRB review of HSR.

The committee found that some nations have adopted laws or regulations that allow individuals to exclude their personally identifiable health information from databases, that require written consent from patients for use of health records for research, and that require the anonymization of data for use in any secondary data analysis. Such measures were enacted to protect privacy and the confidentiality of computerized personally identifiable health information.

If patients and members of the public in general do not find that they can trust that confidential information will be protected throughout research, they may seek further measures to protect confidentiality that could be detrimental to HSR. The committee therefore urges investigators, data users, and data holders and publishers voluntarily to adopt and continually upgrade the best practices of IRBs and other review boards in ensuring the protection of data privacy and confidentiality in HSR.

Recommendation 5-10. All stakeholders in HSR should support strategies to improve the protection of privacy and confidentiality without impeding research.

The committee found it necessary to at least contemplate additional areas for study. Although there was not time in this project to explore wider-ranging ideas, the committee suggests several as potential starting points in a multifaceted strategy to improve the awareness of privacy issues and improve confidentiality protection practices.

• Federal departments including the DHHS could sponsor a conference to include HSR journal editors and editorial boards to consider special issues devoted to data privacy and adoption or strengthening of policies against publishing research without evidence of prior assessment by an IRB or other review board.

• DHHS and other federal departments and agencies, as well as foundations and state and local granting agencies, could consider possible changes in procedure including revising grant application guidelines and contract proposals to include a section on confidentiality protection and to include privacy experts on peer review panels.

• Funders of HSR including DHHS or other federal departments, foundations, accrediting agencies, health maintenance organizations and private companies could consider supporting research on data protection methods.

• Organizations interested in data privacy and high-quality HSR could sponsor a prize competition for best practices in protecting privacy and confidentiality.

The methods of HSR, applied to data previously collected for other purposes, have been useful in discovering and demonstrating systemic effects and population-level trends in the organization and delivery of health services. It is important that we, as a society, continue to have access to such research in order to inform policy making in both private and governmental arenas. At the same time, it is important that we, as a society, protect the privacy of individuals and of vulnerable groups, and the confidentiality of information that patients share with health care providers. As a result of the present study, the committee has concluded that it is possible both to carry out valuable HSR and to protect confidentiality. However, to do so will require adequate funding. Resources are needed to support dedicated, trained IRB members and staff, to establish organizational confidentiality policies and electronic security practices, to educate researchers, and to provide statistical and computer expertise. The true test of our commitment to the twin values of advancing useful knowledge and protecting confidentiality is whether we are willing to make the needed investments to achieve both goals.

1

Introduction

Health services research (HSR), through the analysis of large databases of health information, offers the potential to improve the quality of health care delivery and the effectiveness of health care policies. At the same time, the analysis of personally identifiable health information from many individuals raises concerns about privacy and confidentiality. We need to protect the individual subjects of study (where participation in the study may, but will not necessarily, benefit these subjects) by taking measures that are reliable, but are also compatible with good research that can benefit society as a whole. Ensuring both values is particularly important at this time because of policy debates about health privacy and the confidentiality of computerized health information, and recent criticisms about the effectiveness of institutional review boards (IRBs) in protecting research subjects, although much of the recent criticism has actually focused on clinical trials.[1]

This project charged the Institute of Medicine (IOM) with gathering information on current practices and principles followed by IRBs that review HSR, both under the federal regulations and in privately sponsored studies. In addition, the IOM was asked to recommend, if appropriate, best practices for safeguarding the confidentiality of personally identifiable health information in HSR.

This introductory chapter summarizes the context of the issue of privacy and confidentiality in health services research, including the background of the

---

[1]Regarding policy and confidentiality, see for example Applebaum, 2000; IOM, 1994; NRC 1997; Etzioni, 1999; Gostin and Hadley, 1998; Hanken, 1996; GHPP, 1999; Goldman, 1998. Regarding IRB effectiveness, see for example Brown (OIG), 1998b, 2000; Brainard, 2000; GAO, 1996; Edger and Rothman, 1995.

study, IRBs, HSR and privacy, and the scope and limitations of the current project. This chapter closes with an overview of the remaining chapters of the report. The remaining chapters describe some current and best practices that the committee learned of pertaining to the protection of confidentiality through the application of technology, implementation of informed policies, and training and support of personnel. Finally, the report suggests further steps that would lead to additional improvements in protection of the confidentiality of HSR, while at the time making oversight by IRBs (or other review boards) more effective and efficient. In this report, "effective oversight" includes the idea that the oversight will be trusted throughout our diversified society and reliable and, thus, able to balance societal benefit and individual privacy. Effective oversight will therefore be an efficient means toward allowing valuable HSR to proceed.

PRIVACY AND RESEARCH

Federal policies on the protection of human subjects in all types of research rest on IRB review of the research proposals and protocols, and on obtaining the informed consent of subjects. Both apply somewhat differently in HSR than in clinical research, which increases the scope and complexity of research oversight in general. IRB review is complicated because HSR studies often have characteristics that cause studies not to require full IRB review and discussion. On the other hand, such independent review of these studies may help ensure that confidentiality is adequately protected. The regulations allowing IRBs to exempt studies from full review are described in more detail in Chapter 2. "Exemption" is a formal term in the regulations applied to studies that have such minimal impact on the subjects that no further oversight by an IRB is needed. For situations of somewhat more, but still small, impact, the proposal might receive expedited review from just one or a few members rather than the entire review board. In general, an IRB representative makes the determination of whether a project might be eligible for exemption or expedited review. Informed consent is complicated because many HSR projects involving analysis of personal health data collected previously for another purpose are eligible for waiver of informed consent. Indeed obtaining informed consent is not feasible for many HSR projects.

The methods of HSR are varied and may include not only secondary analysis of previously collected data, but also primary data collection through surveys and interviews. This report focuses on the secondary analysis of data, including personal health information, that have already been collected for some other purpose, because this type of analysis raises the most challenging ethical issues. In research where investigators collect primary data through surveys and interviews, the subject knows that research is being conducted, can find out more about the research, and has an opportunity to decline to participate. By contrast, in secondary analyses of the type described, individuals may not know that they are subjects of research and may not have the opportunity to decline to participate. The researchers also may be unable to identify subjects individually and, thus, unable to contact them for consent. Some people may, however, object if researchers have access to their health information without their knowledge or consent.

The committee recognized that important privacy and confidentiality concerns also arise in other forms of research using previously collected data (e.g., research using archival tissue specimens) and in many types of research in which new data are collected. Each of these areas merits careful study and the dissemination and adoption of best practices for protecting confidentiality. Indeed, the committee affirms that all personally identifiable health information, no matter how it was collected or for what purpose, should be treated so as to respect privacy and maintain confidentiality. This report reflects the committee's specific charge to focus on the analysis of existing data used in HSR after collection for another purpose.

Privacy and Confidentiality

Justice Louis Brandeis' reference to "the right to be left alone" (*Olmstead v. U.S.*, 1928) stands as a vivid and succinct definition of privacy in general, but for the purposes of this study, definitions more focused on information should be considered (Box 1-1).[2]

For the purposes of HSR, privacy can be understood as a person's ability to restrict access to information about him or herself. Privacy is valued because respecting privacy in turn respects the autonomy of persons, protects against surveillance or intrusion, and allows individuals to control the dissemination and use of information about themselves. Privacy fosters and enhances a sense of self and also promotes the development of character traits and close relationships (IOM, 1994). The federal regulations governing human research (45 CFR 46.102 (f)) discuss privacy in the following terms:

> Private information includes information about behavior that occurs in a context in which an individual can reasonably expect that no observation or recording is taking place, and information which has been provided for specific purposes by an individual and which the individual can reasonably expect will not be made public (for example, a medical record). Private information must be individually identifiable (i.e., the identity of the subject is or may readily be ascertained by the investigator or associated with the information) in order for obtaining the information to constitute research involving human subjects.

The regulations thus characterize privacy in terms of the expectations of the persons whose personally identifiable health information is being discussed and stipulate that the information must be specifically associated with the individual in order for the individual to have a legitimate interest in protecting it. Individuals may, however, be harmed or wronged by information associated with them probabalistically as well as specifically identifiable information.

---

[2]Lowrance, 1997; NRC, 1997; Buckovich, et al., 1999; OPRR, 1993; Bradburn, 2000.

Confidentiality refers to controlling access to the information that an individual has already disclosed, for example, a patient to a treating physician or to an insurance company paying for care. Confidentiality is a major expression of respect for persons, the person who has trusted the health care provider with private information in the belief that the information will be guarded appropriately and used only for that person's benefit. Maintaining confidentiality is considered important also because it encourages patients to seek needed care and to discuss sensitive topics candidly with their physicians. If patients do not believe they can trust their health care providers to maintain confidentiality, they may withhold information to the detriment of the best medical judgment and care they might receive. Confidentiality is violated if the person or institution to whom information is disclosed fails to protect it adequately or discloses it inappropriately without the patient's consent. The dilemma about HSR is that personally identifiable health information that is disclosed or collected for one purpose (clinical care, billing, etc.) is then used without consent for a different purpose (improving the state of knowledge to benefit future and current patients).

Confidentiality is also important to the continued success and vitality of the HSR effort. Just as in the case of medical treatment, research subjects may withhold information if they do not have confidence that what they disclose will be protected. Further, it is crucial to the HSR effort that researchers design studies so that the risk of harm to subjects is minimal, in order to allow the protocol to qualify for a waiver of the informed consent requirement. HSR projects often apply methods to large databases of previously collected information where individual informed consent would be impracticable or impossible. The effect of losing the population's trust in confidentiality may have serious repercussions both for the effective quality of medical care and for the quality of medical records research. A 1999 poll by the California HealthCare Foundation (CHCF, 1999) found that approximately one in five respondents believed their personal medical information to have been improperly disclosed by a health care provider, insurance plan, government agency, or employer. Approximately one in

---

BOX 1-1 Definitions about Privacy

- Informational privacy: the right of individuals to control access to, and the use of, information about themselves.
- Data privacy: Informational privacy especially when the information in question is stored in a database.
- Health Information Privacy: Informational privacy especially when the information in question pertains to the health or medical condition of the individual in question.
- Confidentiality: the manner of treating private information, which has been disclosed by the individual subject of the information to a particular person or persons for a specific purpose, such that further disclosure of the information will not be allowed to occur without authorization.

six respondents said they had taken some extra precautions to make sure that medical information about them remained confidential, including paying out of pocket, giving false information, and avoiding care. These figures have been interpreted both as alarmingly large and as reassuringly small. In either case, the numbers do suggest that there is significant potential for the reliability of personally identifiable health information data to decrease if the population's trust that the confidentiality of personally identifiable health information will be maintained decreases.

Benefits and Risks of Harm in Research

All research on human subjects raises ethical concerns because participants in research undergo risks of potential harm primarily, if not solely, for the benefit of others. Balancing benefit and risk of harm is an essential part of the design of any human subjects research. Physicians are familiar with the ethical obligation to balance benefits and risks when providing clinical care. However, in clinical care the patient both directly benefits from interventions and directly accepts the risks. Research, on the other hand, is not intended to benefit the subjects directly, because we actually do not know which treatment is best, so it is even more important in research to ensure that the risks are acceptable in proportion to the likely benefits, and that the risks are minimized. Indeed, these ethical principles are at the core of federal regulations on research human subjects.

Federal Regulations

Federal regulations govern human subjects research when the research is federally supported or regulated (e.g., by the Food and Drug Administration). The body of federal regulations about human subjects protection (45 CFR 46 Subpart A) is called the Common Rule, since it has been adopted "in common" by many federal departments and agencies that are involved in research with human subjects. The Food and Drug Administration (FDA) has adopted similar regulations tailored to its functions (21 CFR 50 and 56) (this report uses the general term "federal regulations" to refer all CFR sections dealing with human subjects protection). In addition, organizations that carry out many projects that are federally funded and involve human subjects can negotiate multiple project assurances (MPAs) with the Office of Human Research Protections (OHRP, formerly the Office for Protection from Research Risks or OPRR). Most organizations holding MPAs agree to carry out all their research according to federal regulations, regardless of whether all the research is intrinsically subject to Common Rule regulation.

In the federal regulations, the IRB of a particular organization is charged with reviewing and approving all research covered by the regulations that is proposed under the auspices of the organization (note, however, that the responsibility for ensuring compliance falls to the organization, not upon the IRB itself). In order to approve research, the IRB must be satisfied that, among other requirements (45 CFR 46.111):

• risks to subjects are minimized and are reasonable in relation to anticipated benefits,
• selection of subjects is equitable,
• informed consent is obtained to the extent required, and
• provisions to protect the privacy of subjects and to maintain the confidentiality of data are adequate.

HEALTH SERVICES RESEARCH

Health services research is the study of the effects of different modes of organization, delivery, and financing of health care services (see Box 1-2). HSR includes studies of the effectiveness of health care interventions in real-world settings, as contrasted with studies of the efficacy[3] of interventions under controlled settings such as a clinical trial.

HSR raises particular issues regarding the protection of human subjects that differ from the problems of clinical research, just as the methods of HSR differ from the methods of clinical research.[4] First, many HSR projects involve minimal risk of harm to subjects, so they may qualify for a waiver of informed consent and individual informed consent is often impractical or impossible in HSR projects.[5] For example, an HSR project may carry out secondary analyses of data previously collected in the delivery of patient care or the payment for such care. If the subjects whom the project will involve are enrollees in the federal Medicare program, the number of subjects may be as many as several million individuals. Further, many HSR projects use data that are already public and de-identified, so they may qualify for exemption from IRB review or for expedited review. Finally, many private organizations do HSR—or programs such as quality improvement that use similar data and methods—not covered by the federal regulations. These organizations may not have IRBs.

---

[3]The term "efficacy" refers to how reliably an intervention brings about a given result under ideal, controlled conditions. The term "effectiveness" refers to how an intervention performs in the complex and variable context of real-world use and practice.

[4]There are other fields of research such as epidemiology, however, that share with HSR similar methods and databases but evaluate different public health questions, (e.g. the frequency of rare medication side effects). Although not examined here, the practices reviewed by the committee for HSR would likely apply in these other fields.

[5]Informed consent is not always feasible for clinical trials either: FDA regulations at 21 CFR 50.24 allow for the use of investigational drugs without informed consent under certain conditions such as cases where the subject's condition is immediately life-threatening, the subject is not able to participate in giving consent, time does not permit seeking proxy consent, and no alternative approved or generally recognized therapy is available.

Since the object of HSR includes the study of health care operations and HSR uses many of the same methods used in health care operations units to assess their own performance, HSR is fundamentally connected to nonresearch investigations within heath care organizations.

The committee heard one account describing the situation as a continuum, with HSR at one end of the scale and operations at the other end (see Figure 3 in Appendix B). Some HSR projects are clear examples of research; applying scientific methods to test hypotheses and produce new, generalizable knowledge. Other projects are certainly clear examples of internal exercises to assess the quality of the operations of the specific organization with no intention of producing generalizable knowledge. At the same time, quality assessment and quality improvement (QA and QI) exercises sometimes reveal interesting and important data that the organization recognizes to be of general interest, and that therefore ought to be published. In addition, both scientific research in health services and investigations into the internal operation of a health services organization use many of the same methods (e.g., chart review, database analysis and linkage).

In fact, many projects may start out as operations assessment and then become more like research, and many research projects involve doing very much what would be done in an internal operations assessment. This continuum is one of the interesting, if problematic, features of HSR. The committee proceeded with a view to the clearer cases of research in health services, always mindful of the less clear cases and closely related operations assessment exercises. From the point of view of the patient or subject—the person whose personally identifiable health information may be reviewed or used—the continuum appears more like a widening circle of disclosure. At the center is the individual and health information not yet shared with anyone; then, according to Etzioni's description (Etzioni, 1999), comes the inner circle of those with whom the individual shares information because they will use the information directly in the care

---

BOX 1-2 Definitions of Health Services Research

Institute of Medicine, (IOM):

Health services research is a multidisciplinary field of inquiry, both basic and applied, that examines the use, costs, quality, accessibility, delivery, organization, financing, and outcomes of health care services to increase knowledge and understanding of the structure, processes, and effects of health services for individuals and populations.

Association for Health Services Research:

Health Services Research is a field of inquiry using quantitative or qualitative methodology to examine the impact of the organization, financing and management of health care services on the access to, delivery, cost, outcomes and quality of services.

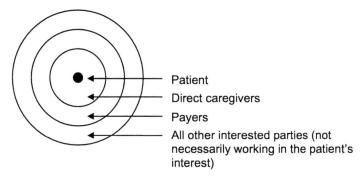

Patient
Direct caregivers
Payers
All other interested parties (not
necessarily working in the patient's
interest)

FIGURE 1-1 Circles of disclosure. SOURCE: Adapted from Etzioni 1999.

of that individual. Next comes the intermediate circle of payers, and finally the widest circle of everyone else who may have an interest in the individual's health information (but with whom the individual may or may not have an interest in sharing the information [Figure 1-1]).

The clearest examples of QA and QI occur in organizations involved in health care delivery or payment. In many such assessments, individual patient cases have to be reviewed. For example, if an organization is trying to reduce drug errors in the hospital or shorten the length of stay after coronary bypass surgery, for example, it may need to review the medical records of individual patients to get a clear idea of how the process of care might be improved. Furthermore, when a health care organization is investigating a "critical incident" in which an error occurred, the QA committee will have to review the individual case in detail. HSR studies generally do not require investigators to know all personal information about each individual subject, but they often do require preservation of linkages (via consistent code numbers) across data files for individuals.

BENEFITS OF HSR

HSR can lead to improvements in the delivery and organization of health care, which may in turn improve health outcomes, and the cost-effectiveness of care, for patients. It addresses large-scale systemic effects of health care delivery changes that are difficult if not impossible to understand at the level of the individual citizen, consumer, or patient. This kind of information is important for planners and policy developers in both government and the health care industry. It is also increasingly important for both corporate and individual consumers of health care services (Clancy and Eisenberg, 1998; Eisenberg, 1998). Our health care system is incorporating greater reliance on market decisions to improve quality and control costs, but these decisions can be made well only with access to good information about different health care services options. HSR provides objective data on questions about the effectiveness of institutional variables, just as clinical trials assess the efficacy of interventions in individuals. HSR projects aim at a variety of levels of the health care system. Some examples follow.

Policy Assessment   Well-intentioned public policies may have unanticipated adverse consequences or fail to fulfill their goals. However, whether they are meeting or missing their goals, it is often difficult to assess their outcomes without a systematic examination. HSR generates data on the outcomes of public policies and provides an empirical base for modification or refinement of these policies. For example, Gross et al. (1998) compared previously collected data from several sources (including the Medicare Current Beneficiary Survey) to estimate out-of-pocket health care spending by lower-income Medicare beneficiaries. The authors found that although Medicaid provides significant protection for some lower-income Medicare beneficiaries, out-of-pocket health care spending continues to be a substantial burden for most of this population. This fact may be important in considering policies that would depend on further cost shifting to increase out-of-pocket expenditure. In another example, Cromwell et al. (1998) compared data over a four-year period on Medicaid anti-ulcer drug claims, Medicaid eligibility, and acute care nonfederal hospital discharges to assess what effect a policy of restricting reimbursement for Medicaid anti-ulcer drugs had on the use of these drugs and on peptic ulcer-related hospitalizations. Following implementation of the policy, reimbursements for the drugs decreased 33 percent but there was no associated increase in the rate of Medicaid peptic ulcer-related hospitalizations. These results opened further research questions because there may have been quality-of-life implications for some patients that the study did not address. Addressing these questions has important public policy implications.

Outcome Predictors   The question of whether it makes a difference to have a procedure done in a hospital that has a high case load of similar procedures is important to policy makers and to individuals who may need an operation. HSR studies have demonstrated in several cases that centers performing a greater volume of procedures have better patient outcomes. Norton et al. (1998) examined the effects of case volume on outcomes for knee replacement surgery using Medicare claims data and found the results so striking that they recommended against expanding knee replacement surgery to new centers generally and instead recommended concentrating on developing hub centers. Other groups of investigators have examined the relationship between volume and outcomes in coronary interventions, where the inverse relation between volume and mortality has been known for two decades. This does not mean that new information is not important in changing policy, however. Sollano et al. (1999) investigated the outcomes in several New York hospitals of three types of operations and found that although the relationship (high volume associated with lower mortality) persisted in two, it no longer held true for the third, coronary artery bypass grafting. The authors attribute the disappearance of the relationship in this operation to a recent quality improvement program in bypass operations in the region, with important implications for the effects of QI programs in general. On a similar note, Malenka et al. (1999) showed that for one type of surgery (percutaneous coronary interventions), the operator did not have to do as many procedures per year to maintain top performance as had previously been believed, which they attributed to changes in practice due to new devices and drugs.

Provider Practices HSR develops data on physician behavior and practices. Zito et al. (2000) recently demonstrated a significant overall increase in the rate of prescriptions of psychotropic drugs for preschool-aged children (using data from two state Medicaid programs and a salaried group-model health maintenance organization [HMO]), which is of note in part because there are few controlled clinical trials of the safety and efficacy of such drugs in this young age group.

HSR studies also help identify factors that may predict underuse of services that are known to be beneficial. HSR has shown that patients who have survived one heart attack also are known to have lower mortality if they receive medications such as beta-blockers, aspirin, and cholesterol-lowering drugs, yet these drugs are underused. Recent research confirms this and supports the use of beta-blockers even in diabetic patients, a group for whom some physicians had been reluctant to prescribe them (Chen et al., 1999). Other HSR studies have sought to address questions of the adoption or lack of adoption of clinical practice guidelines. Katz (1998) found, on analyzing the AHRQ guideline for unstable angina, that there were several barriers to adoption including physician variability. These included incomplete specification of exceptions as well as unexpected increases in demand for care. Recognition of these barriers can then be incorporated in the development of future guidelines to ease their adoption.

Effects of Business Practices and Law on Health Product Delivery Brooks et al. (1998) used HSR techniques to demonstrate that independent pharmacies are at significant disadvantage compared to chains when negotiating with insurers. Collective bargaining by pharmacies might mitigate this disadvantage but is currently prevented by antitrust law. Such information would be impossible for a consumer to obtain and therefore impossible to act on, yet the consumer certainly feels the effects on the pocket book of more or less negotiating power.

RISKS OF HARM FROM HSR

The risks of HSR are primarily violations of privacy and confidentiality, not physical risks. HSR thus differs from clinical research in which patients are at risk for physical harms because they undergo invasive medical procedures or receive unproven new therapies. Potential risks of violations of privacy or breaches of confidentiality are by no means limited to research, but can occur anytime personally identifiable health information has been collected. Potential risks include the following:

• Risk of public (or private) disclosure of protected health secrets, which can lead to stigmatization or discrimination in employment or insurance, and/or shame: this is the fundamental issue and, for most people, probably the most serious.

• Risk of disruption of, or interference in, patterns within families, which may result from unexpected and unauthorized communication of secrets within the family.

• Risk that individuals may recognize (correctly or not) their own health history or anecdotes in results and interpretations of a study or may suffer anxiety simply from knowing that personal data may be in a database, without knowing whether adequate privacy protections are in place: this subjects the person to the *perception* of the first risk, even if it is not actually present.

• Risk of future contact. Privacy is "the right to be left alone." Yet some HSR studies permit the collection of follow-up investigations that include contacting the individual whose data are studied. In this case, a stranger to the person or (perhaps less alarming but still disruptive) a care provider from long ago can suddenly intrude upon the subject's right to be left alone.

• Risk of loss of trust in the health care system and/or scientific research, and thus loss of willingness to participate in future studies or perhaps even to seek needed health care.[6]

These psychosocial harms can be avoided or mitigated if the research data are coded or encrypted in such a way that individual subjects cannot be identified. In addition, some harms can be prevented by strong antidiscrimination laws. However, subjects may be *wronged* by violations of privacy and confidentiality, even if they suffer no tangible harm. That is, even if persons do not suffer employment difficulties or can be compensated by law if they do, this does not change the fact that the subjects did not receive the respect due them as persons. The federal regulations on research on human subjects explicitly require IRBs to consider wrongs as well as harms in assessing the benefits and risks of research.

Breaches in the confidentiality of previously collected data can occur in a variety of ways. For example, an employee who has a legitimate need to access part of the database to carry out his or her job may make unauthorized use of that access: a clerk in charge of determining insurance eligibility, or a nurse who is not providing direct care to the patient, may review the records of an acquaintance or a celebrity just for the sake of satisfying curiosity. The great majority of occasions for data transfer and access occur not through research (or malfeasance), but in standard health care operations. The great majority of occasions for breach of confidentiality likewise occur in daily operations.[7] Some instances of breaches of confidentiality are unintentional, for example, leaving a record that includes a patient's name out in the view of a visitor or discussing a

---

[6]For a full discussion of this problem see, for example, Goldman (1998).

[7]The recent NRC report *For the Record* (1997) discussed the increasing complexity of health information flow in detail (see especially Figure 3.1) p. 73. See also Goldman and Hudson (1999).

patient by name in the hearing of other parties in an elevator or cafeteria (Ubel et al., 1995).[8] Also, some breaches are not accidental, but are oversights. The committee heard of one incident in which the names of employees tested for HIV were displayed with the test results on a slide at a presentation, for example. The aim of the presentation was simply to describe a database of in-house health records. Some of the employees whose records were listed in the section displayed were actually attending the meeting. In this case the breach of confidentiality could have been avoided through more attention or training on the part of the research team and by the use of coded identifiers rather than direct identifiers such as names.

As our health care system becomes more complex, information flow is likewise increasingly complicated and the potential occasions for either a breach, or perception of a breach, of confidentiality are correspondingly multiplied. For example, a database marketing firm received patient prescription records from two large pharmacies in the Washington, D.C. metro area (Lo and Alpers, 2000). The firm then created mailings targeted to consumers of certain prescription drug products on behalf of the pharmacies (using the letterhead of the pharmacies), informing them of new products with similar indications. The project was sponsored by the manufacturers of the new products, though the manufacturers did not have access to patient data. Many of the recipients were disturbed at receiving the letters, since the action seemed to straddle or even cross the line between standard prescription medication compliance letters that are often sent by pharmacies to patients and product marketing.[9]

Despite the potential for misuse, there are important and legitimate reasons to maintain some identifiability in personal health information databases. Much of the value of retrospective data-based research comes from the ability to draw

---

[8]In some cases the disclosure may be intentional: a particularly famous example of the improper disclosure of personally identifiable health information occurred with the unauthorized release of the HIV status of Mr. Arthur Ashe (mentioned widely, e.g., in Shalala, 1997). It is important in the context of this report, however, to note that this disclosure was not made in the course of research, and it was accomplished with paper records. Of course, such disclosures are also not part of *normal* health care operations.

[9]Perceptions of breach of confidentiality can also include cases where an individual has (knowingly or unknowingly) provided information in the course of responding to a consumer survey or calling a product hotline, either of which often results in the individual receiving marketing materials including disease-related product advertising information. On receiving such information, some individuals may assume that private health information was shared by their health care providers, not realizing that they themselves had provided the information for the marketing effort. A different type of concern, again not in research but in operations, was described in a previous IOM report, *Health Data in the Information Age* (IOM, 1994). The report noted that increasing the fringe benefits offered by employers also increases pressure on the employers to control costs and that information about an employee's health may be shared through the company to tailor plans so as to reduce liability (the report referred to a case that upheld the right of an employer to reduce benefits, in which an employer became self-insured and established a limit on AIDS-related expenses after a current employee was diagnosed with AIDS [p. 159]).

inferences from data derived from different sources. For example, health care organizations are often interested in identifying episodes of illness in a patient, which may be manifest in records of emergency room visits, ambulance services, hospital stays, operative records, bills from independent medical providers, rehabilitation services, pharmacies and pharmacy benefit managers, and so forth. In order to recognize that the data drawn from these various sources refer to the experiences of a single individual, it is important that researchers be able to identify the same patient in each set of records. This identification allows joining these various datasets into a single (logical) database that contains all relevant data about the patient. Such identification and joining is often difficult, and is one of the motivations for keeping identifiers. The actual identity of any individual is not really necessary to support the linkage between databases that have been joined; all that is required is a unique identifier, which might (at least in principle) be difficult to re-associate with the actual patient.

Even when research data are recorded in coded or encrypted format, however, it may be possible to identify individual subjects at least with good probability. Records are directly identifiable when individual identifiers such as names or Social Security numbers are collected or retained (also called "manifest identifiability"). Yet individuals might be identified, at least probabilistically, by linking otherwise de-identified data so that the resulting record effectively identifies a particular individual. In this latter case, the information is said to be indirectly identifiable (or "identifiable by inference"). For example, race may not be a direct or manifest identifier in the general population, but when combined with the zip code of a relatively homogeneous area, a person of contrasting race could be identified.

In one example of identification by inference, Latanya Sweeney showed that three data fields (e.g., birth date, sex, and zip code) were sufficient to create a linkage in databases, locating, with good probability, the records pertaining to a single individual who was employed by the state. She was able to do this a matter of hours using data that had been made publicly available only after all the (known) identifiers had been removed (L. Sweeney, personal communication, 2000; Sweeney in press; see also Sweeney, 1997, for further discussion). This example shows, first, that supposedly de-identified data may still be personally identifiable when combined with other available data that either are complete or do identify individuals. Second, it shows that the ability to manipulate databases to locate individual subjects has increased due to advances in computing. Even if the information collected is no more invasive now than previously, it is now feasible for others to glean personally identifiable health information from such data where it would have been much more difficult before.

Sweeney's demonstration should be a reminder that with the increasing technical ease of identification by inference, there can be no guarantee of absolute confidentiality of records. This fact in turn raises the question of how much effort and expense ought reasonably to be invested in privacy protection. There are various approaches to minimizing breaches of confidentiality. Some call for strong measures at the point of disclosure, such as increasing the types of disclosures where explicit informed consent would be required (Norsigian and Billings, 1998; Woodward, 1999); others emphasize strong sanctions against violations of confidentiality by the data holders or users who release or receive secondary data; and finally, still others argue that the best course would be to stop worrying about it entirely and instead turn to developing ways to live in society without informational barriers (as suggested by the now-well-known aphorism of Sun Microsystem's corporate executive officer Scott McNealy, "There is no privacy, get over it").

There are several important points to keep in mind about the risk of breaches in confidentiality: the risk is neither new nor research specific, and some level of risk is inevitable. First, the improper identification and disclosure of health information about individuals is not a unique risk from HSR, nor is it a new result of the widespread adoption of computer-based patient records, governmental or health care industry databases or the Internet. Most instances occur outside of research, in operations. Also, breaches occurred with paper records as well. It is the case, however, that with the development of computing and communications technology, both intentional and unintentional identification and disclosure of electronic personally identifiable health information potentially involve more types of information and more individuals than were possible with paper records. At the most basic level, confidentiality always depends on conscious efforts by human agents to treat other human beings with respect and restraint, whether the activity is research or not, and whatever the state of the technology.

The protection of confidentiality is impossible to guarantee—some level of risk is inevitable.[10] It is possible to make breaches less likely and to increase the probability that confidentiality will be maintained, but the protection of confidentiality is a matter of shifting the probabilities; it cannot be an absolute (see also GHPP, 1999, pp. 15–16). The question really is what measures can be taken to enhance confidentiality protection, and thus retain public trust in HSR, and

---

[10]The probabilistic nature of confidentiality has been recognized elsewhere, for instance a 1998 working group convened by the National Cancer Institute of the National Institute of Health to examine the creation of informed consent documents had the following recommendation regarding informing potential subjects about confidentiality and its limitations:

> Confidentiality: The confidentiality section of the informed consent document should state that although measures will be taken to protect the privacy and security of personally-identifiable data, absolute confidentiality cannot be guaranteed. The consent document should list the organizations that will have access to personally-identifiable data and that personally identifiable information may be disclosed as required by law. When listing organizations that will have access to research records, describe for what purposes the information will be disclosed to these organizations. (From Recommendations for the Development of Informed Consent Documents for Cancer Clinical Trials, by the Comprehensive Working Group on Informed Consent in Cancer Clinical Trials for the National Cancer Institute, October 1998, posted at the following address, http://cancertrials.nci.nih.gov/researchers/safeguards/consent/recs.html#Confidentiality).

still allow research to proceed. Since it is not possible to guarantee the confidentiality of records in general, it is also not possible to guarantee absolute confidentiality in HSR. The measures we can take to increase the protection of privacy and confidentiality are varied, some simple and some complex, and the range of measures will change as computational and communications technologies develop. The committee argues that with appropriate safeguards for confidentiality, it is acceptable to consider a great deal of HSR as minimal risk and appropriate to carry out without requesting consent for each reanalysis of data.

BACKGROUND AND POLICY CONTEXT

In recent years, public concern about privacy and maintaining the confidentiality of personally identifiable health information has increased. Legislators have responded to worried constituents by introducing a variety of privacy bills over several sessions of Congress. Currently, there is no comprehensive federal law that protects privacy for all health-related information. There are some federal, and varying state, statutes that protect certain types of personally identifiable health information under certain circumstances (see, e.g., Gostin, et al, 1996; O'Brian and Yasnoff; 1999, also Pritts et al., 1999). One state action that has generated considerable interest of late was the Minnesota Access to Health Records Law (McCarthy et al., 1999), which required informed consent from patients to use of their medical records for research. There has been disagreement as to the actual intent and effect of this law (Melton, 1997; Norsigian and Billings, 1998). Whatever the law's actual impact, it expresses public concerns about privacy in research. The committee felt that these concerns were important to address through effective privacy and confidentiality protections and also believed that good protection could be implemented so as to be compatible with future research. The committee hopes that this report will help address these concerns (see Box 1-3 for more definitions).

In 1996, Congress enacted the Health Insurance Portability and Accountability Act (HIPAA), directing the Secretary of Health and Human Services to create detailed recommendations on standards with respect to the privacy of personally identifiable health information. The Secretary's recommendations were delivered to Congress in September 1997 (Shalala, 1997), and several privacy bills have been introduced in Congress since. Both the Secretary's recommendations and most of the privacy bills introduced in the 105th Congress would permit research using personally identifiable health information without the subject's explicit permission if the research project were approved by an institutional review board.

The HIPAA further directed the Secretary of Health and Human Services to create regulations by February 2000, unless the Congress had taken legislative action at least six months earlier. Congress did not take further action, so the

BOX 1-3 More Definitions

Common Rule—the central federal policy adopted "in common" by 16 federal departments and agencies (and concurred, with some modifications, by the FDA) that support and/or conduct research involving human subjects. The adoption of the federal policy in 1991 implements a recommendation of the President's Commission for the Study of Ethical Problems in Medicine and Biomedical and Behavioral Research that all federal departments and agencies "adopt as a common core the regulations governing research with human subjects issued by the Department of Health and Human Services (codified at 45 CFR 46, Subpart A), as periodically amended or revised, while permitting additions needed by any department or agency that are not inconsistent with these core provisions" (OPRR Guidebook, Chapter 2).

(Federal) Regulations—Regulations are the rules that departments or agencies issue to provide specific guidance to themselves and others about how they will implement pertinent laws. In this particular report, "regulations" refers to federal regulations on human subjects protection implementing the Common Rule. This report usually provides the citation to the DHHS regulations, since that agency sponsors most of the relevant research and this project, but the report applies similarly to other departments and agencies.

Personally Identifiable Health Information—Health or medical data or information that can be linked manifestly or inferentially to an individual.

The terms "anonymized" and "de-identified" are commonly used to refer to health information where some attempt has been made to provide confidentiality protections by making it difficult to link a record to a specific individual. An additional difficulty, as discussed in the text, is that the ability to re-identify an individual from a dataset depends not only on the degree to which identity is hidden or removed in that dataset, but also on access to other datasets that may facilitate probabilistic identification of the individual. It is thus very difficult for anyone to assure anonymity of a dataset because critical factors in re-identifiability depend on conditions outside the dataset. The terms "anonymized" and "de-identified" exist along a spectrum of properties of data and are not guaranteed endpoints (GHPP, 1999). Since people do not always specify what they mean by these terms, individuals may define them in different ways. The committee suggests:

> *De-Identified*—Refers to information or data where direct identifiers such as name and address have been removed. In common use the term refers to data where it may still be possible to identify individuals by inference or through codes held by the investigator or a third party. Therefore data that is *de-identified* may not be *anonymized* because it may still permit at least probabilistic re-identification when analyzed in conjunction with other datasets.

Continued

BOX 1-3 *Continued*

Anonymized—Refers to information or data where identifiers (and codes that are linked to identifiers) have been removed, as well as other values that would enable individuals to be identified by inference. Close correlation with values in additional datasets, or unique values, or cells containing few data points, for instance, could support such inferences. A dataset, therefore, must at least have been thoroughly de-identified in order to be anonymized. For all practical purposes, anonymized data cannot be linked to the individual. Examples of anonymized data are public use files made available by the Bureau of the Census.

The DHHS proposal would create new requirements for privacy protection for all health care providers and health plans, and would establish research standards and oversight for all research. The proposed regulations suggest that the review function be performed by boards that are equipped to deal with data privacy and by organizational privacy officers who will ensure system-wide compliance with new privacy rules. The proposed regulations contemplate that IRBs might conduct privacy review in some circumstances, but the DHHS proposal does not suggest that IRBs are the only or even the best mechanism for privacy review with respect to data studies. The proposed rule would permit the use and disclosure of personally identifiable health information for research without authorization by the subject, as long as the research protocol had been approved by an IRB established in accord with the Common Rule (or FDA regulations) or by a privacy board. The proposed rule then specifies that a privacy board would have to have members with varying backgrounds but appropriate professional competence, at least one member not affiliated with the organization doing the research, and no members with conflicts of interest (DHHS, 1999, p. 60058).[11] As this report was being written, DHHS was analyzing and responding to the approximately 52,000 comments that the proposed rule elicited. Recent studies of IRBs are another important policy context for this report: several have questioned whether IRBs adequately fulfill their role of protecting research subjects and whether they have sufficient resources to do so.

---

[11]The preamble to the proposed rule further specifies a privacy board as a body equivalent to an IRB. During the comment period, various parties disagreed about whether the privacy board as specified would actually be equivalent to an IRB and able to provide the degree of oversight necessary.

Historically, the focus of IRBs has been on protecting human subjects from potential harm associated with participation in clinical research that involves invasive medical procedures or new drugs. Little is known about IRB practices in the area of HSR projects, though DHHS regulations at 45 CFR 46 have always applied to non-clinical, as well as to clinical, research. Furthermore, much HSR using large databases is undertaken with private funding and, consequently, falls outside the purview of IRBs.

PROJECT AND SCOPE

This report is the product of a project sponsored by two agencies within the DHHS, the Agency for Healthcare Research and Quality (AHRQ) and the Office of the Assistant Secretary for Planning and Evaluation (ASPE).

This report is intended for all types of professionals and organizations that use or disclose data on health services. For organizations that have IRBs whose research is subject to federal regulation, the recommendations highlight practices already in place in some IRBs and suggest additional support for IRB activities. For organizations that use or disclose data but do not have an IRB or whose work is not subject to federal regulation, the practices and recommendations emphasize that the protection of human subjects from risks, including nonphysical risks from use of data, is of concern to anyone who uses or discloses data.
that the protection of of human subjects from risks, including nonphysical risks form use of data, is of concern to to anyone who uses or discloses data.

Although not all organizations have IRBs, all human subjects should be treated with the same high standards. The committee urges organizations that do not have IRBs to adopt practices of reviewing proposed investigations to ensure that data confidentiality will be maintained. The committee likewise urges organizations that have, as well as those that do not have, IRBs to adopt system-wide confidentiality procedures and policies to protect nonresearch and research data.

The purpose of this project was to provide information and advice to the sponsors on the current and best practices of IRBs in protecting privacy in HSR. The charge to the committee was given in three parts as shown below.

1. To gather information on the current practices and principles followed by IRBs to safeguard the confidentiality of personally identifiable health information used for health services research purposes, in particular, to identify those IRB practices that are superior in protecting the privacy, confidentiality, and security of personally identifiable health information.

2. To gather information on the current practices and principles employed in privately funded health services research studies (that are generally not subject to IRB approval) to safeguard the confidentiality of personally identifiable health information, and to consider whether and how IRB best practices in this regard might be applied to such privately sponsored studies.

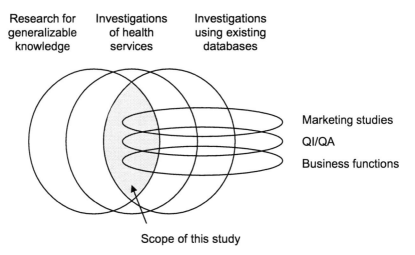

FIGURE 1-2 Scope of the Institute of Medicine study.

3. If appropriate, to recommend a set of best practices for safeguarding the confidentiality of personally identifiable health information that might be voluntarily applied to health services research projects by IRBs and private sponsors.

In order to address these tasks, the IOM assembled a 12-member committee with expertise in medical ethics, health services research, IRB function, statistics, computer science, law, and database management. The committee met by telephone conference in January 2000. The committee and the IOM then convened a public workshop in March 2000. The committee invited testimony from IRB chairs and administrators, health services researchers, and other officers of academia, government and private industry (see Appendix B). The workshop also featured presentations of the drafts of two commissioned papers, one addressing special considerations of health services research and confidentiality when the data pertain to minors (see Appendix C) and the other presenting an international comparison of health information privacy standards (see Appendix D). In addition to the workshop, the committee posted an invitation on a list serve and on the National Academies' website to IRBs to contribute information (see Appendix A). The committee collected further information informally by e-mail and telephone. The committee deliberated by telephone and e-mail, and in a closed meeting in April 2000, about the practices described to it. Finally the committee has summarized the practices it heard that seemed to be most effective in this report.

The committee addressed privacy and confidentiality pertaining to data used in health services research that had already been collected for another purpose. There are many other aspects of the privacy of electronic medical records that were beyond the charge to the committee (Figure 1-2). The committee focused its work on secondary analyses of data that had already been collected for other uses, because such studies pose the most difficult ethical issues regarding HSR.

Although HSR that utilizes surveys and interviews (including the qualitative HSR mentioned in Box 1-2) also raises ethical issues, the contact between researchers and subjects allows the subjects to learn about the research and decline to participate if they so choose. The committee recognized the strong connections between these related matters and the question of protecting data privacy in health services research that uses existing data. The committee therefore asks the reader to bear in mind that such related matters were not in its charge, were not addressed by the committee, and in particular, were not discussed at the workshop.

OUTLINE OF REPORT

Chapter 2 summarizes the federal regulations as they apply to HSR studies. Chapter 3 presents the committee's recommendations and findings based on the available information from IRB's working under federal regulations. Chapter 4 presents the committee's recommendations and findings based on available information from health care services and products companies that may not have IRBs or be subject to federal regulations. The committee holds the conviction that studies involving human subjects should be reviewed similarly whether the study is subject to Common Rule provisions or not. As a result, the committee makes similar recommendations regarding research that falls under the Common Rule and research that does not. The committee considered combining chapters 3 and 4, but decided to keep them separate both because the implications of the recommendations might be different for different types or organizations, and because the separate structure seemed to reflect the committee's charge more clearly. Finally, Chapter 5 returns to the topic of the limited scope of this project in discussing research and steps for the future. As was mentioned in the workshop, the end of this study must not be the end of studying these important questions, and the final chapter suggests some directions for further work.

The committee gathered information through a public workshop (summarized in Appendix B), a general information request posted through the internet (see Appendix A), and various unstructured interviews in the course of study operations. Although the committee received just a few responses to the posted call for information, those received were very informative. The committee noted that all the providers of information, including respondents to the call for information, those who briefed the staff by telephone, and participants in the workshop, are a self-selected group of professionals committed to the IRB process. Information collection was thus not systematic and random, but particularly targeted. The committee also commissioned two background papers, one to examine HSR and minors and the other to compare privacy and confidentiality standards across national borders, which appear as Appendixes C and D. Finally, biographical sketches of the committee members are included as Appendix E.

2

Human Subjects Protection and Health Services Research in Federal Regulations

This chapter presents a brief summary of the federal regulations governing the protection of human subjects in research, with particular attention to how the concepts of the regulations fit with the methodology of health services research (HSR). It provides background for the chapters on the practices of organizations involved in human subjects research, since one of the primary goals of this project is to help understand how institutional review boards (IRBs) implement these regulations for HSR.

IRBs AND HUMAN SUBJECTS PROTECTION

The cornerstones of U.S. regulations on the protection of human subjects are review by institutional review boards and informed consent from participants in research.

Background of Federal Regulations

The Belmont Report (Belmont, 1979) articulated three principles for research on human subjects: *respect for persons, beneficence,* and *justice.* "Respect for persons," in the analysis of the report, includes the notions that each human individual should be treated as an autonomous agent and that those whose capacities preclude autonomy either temporarily or throughout life are owed special protection. The main practical expression of the principle of respect for persons is the requirement that the researcher first obtain the informed consent of the subject(s). "Beneficence," or doing good, requires that the risks of research be reasonable in relation to the possible benefits and that any risks subjects may incur be minimized.[1] "Justice" requires that benefits and harms of research be shared fairly. Applying the justice principle, the IRB should ensure that the selection of subjects or potential subject populations is equitable. Of course it is one thing to enunciate general principles and quite another to ensure their consistent and correct application in particular cases. There are many difficult borderline issues in the ethics of human subjects research. Difficulties in applying the principles underlying regulations on the protection of human subjects in HSR differ from those in clinical research (Iezzoni, 1999 and Lo, 1999). These difficulties stem, in large part, from the history of the documents articulating human subjects protection and the nature and methodology of HSR federal regulations assume that clinical research is the paradigmatic use of human subjects and therefore are directed primarily toward avoiding physical harm to the individual subject. HSR studies, however, are generally more removed from the human subjects, because they employ methodologies for sorting, linking, and otherwise manipulating previously collected data. This aspect of HSR raises a variety of questions about application of the ethical principles underlying our beliefs about the proper treatment of human subjects. The question of whether a particular project is research can have substantial ramifications in the ethical, scientific, legal, and procedural requirements attached to it (Lo, 1999).

IRB Review

In the United States, federally supported and regulated human subjects research is covered by regulations adopted specifically by 16 federal agencies that conduct, support, or regulate research with human subjects. This shared body of regulation, which is the "Common Rule," appears at 45 CFR 46 Subpart A for the Department of Health and Human Services. The Food and Drug Administration has adopted similar regulations at 21 CFR 50 and 56.

IRB review ensures that the proposed research protocol will be reviewed by people who are knowledgeable and not directly involved in the research. The IRB's membership and function are defined in the regulations to ensure that it has sufficient expertise and diversity to provide appropriate review. Diversity

---

[1]It is important to realize that this requirement is not redundant. The first part considers the relative benefits and risks of a protocol, and acknowledges that increased scientific understanding is desirable but is completely without cost. At the same time, the second part mandates that an overall benefit–risk calculation ought not be made without simultaneously considering the cost to the individual. That is, making the benefit–risk calculation in part 1 of the requirement treats the subject as a *means* to realizing a benefit. The part 2 provides a check on part 1, ensuring that the subject is not treated as a means *only*. The lack of the part 2 check is why there has been controversy about using the results of certain Nazi experiments, notably the series on hypothermia: the data may be sound, but even if the information gained would benefit society, the cost to the subjects was unacceptable, so many regard the data as tainted beyond redemption (Ivy, 1947, in Reiser et al., 1977).

should include gender, race, culture, and profession. In addition to scientists, the IRB must include at least one person who is not otherwise connected with the institution and at least one non-scientist.

Many factors must be considered in evaluating the risks and benefits of a research project, including its scientific merit and policy relevance, its relevance to the local community, community values and standards of care, the specific research setting, the populations targeted for recruitment, the nature of the research questions and measures, and the cultural diversity of the target populations. For these reasons, a good IRB needs to have experts both with local and with national knowledge.

What Research Is Subject to Federal Regulations?

Federal regulations apply to all research involving human subjects that is supported by federal funds, with certain exceptions. In addition, the FDA has a policy of not reviewing any research submitted with a new product application unless that research was conducted according to the regulations, regardless of funding (21 CFR 56.103(a) and (b); see also, for example regarding contents of applications to investigate or market new drugs, 21 CFR 312.66 and 314.50(d)(3)(i)).

Many organizations that conduct a great deal of federally funded or regulated research involving human subjects have multiple project assurances (MPAs) through the Office of Human Research Protections (OHRP, formerly Office for Protection from Research Risks or OPRR) in which they have agreed to comply with federal regulations for any human subjects research, even those projects that are funded by some non-federal source and would not otherwise to covered by the regulations. An "assurance" is an agreement or contract between an institution and the OHRP, on behalf of the Secretary of Health and Human Services. The assurance stipulates the methods by which the institution will protect the rights and welfare of research subjects in accordance with the regulations. An MPA can be approved for up to five-year intervals.[2]

What Establishes a Project as Research?

The definition of research in the regulations specifies "a systematic investigation . . . designed to develop or contribute to generalizable knowledge" (45 CFR 46.102(d)). As discussed in the committee's workshop (see appendix B), the

---

[2]MPA is defined in the OPRR Guidebook Chapter 2, Section A(iii). There are several thousand IRBs in operation, though estimates of the exact number vary between 3,000 and 5,000 (OIG, 2000, p. 20). Approximately 750 of these IRBs are located in approximately 430 organizations (some have several IRBs) that have entered into MPAs with the OHRP. The great majority (more than 98 percent) of these MPAs cover all human subjects research in the organization, although a few organizations have limited their MPAs to cover only federally funded studies (Gary Ellis, formerly of OPRR, and Jon Merz, University of Pennsylvania, personal communications).

interpretation of the key phrase "generalizable knowledge" is difficult and can be controversial.[3] Some IRBs interpret this phrase to cover only projects in which the investigator intends to publish the results, whereas others interpret the phrase as covering projects whose results are disseminated beyond the department or unit conducting the study, for example, dissemination through oral presentations at scientific or other professional meetings. The difficulty is especially acute in defining the boundaries of HSR since, as discussed in the previous chapter, many projects could reasonably be categorized either as research "designed to contribute to generalizable knowledge" or as "as internal quality assurance."

What Establishes a Research Study as Involving Human Subjects?

The regulations define a human subject as "a living individual about whom an investigator conducting research obtains data through intervention or interaction with the individual, or identifiable private information (45 CFR 46.102(f)). The former is not applicable in studies analyzing previously collected data. Private information, in this context, is defined as "information about behavior that occurs in a context in which an individual can reasonably expect that no observation or recording is taking place, and information which has been provided for specific purposes by an individual and which the individual can reasonably expect will not be made public (e.g., a medical record) (45 CFR 46.102(f)). The definition stipulates that the information must be individually identifiable, that is, the identity of the individual can readily be ascertained or associated with the information. In short, the open question for a project in HSR is whether the information is identifiable.

What HSR May Be Exempt from IRB Review?

The regulations allow an IRB to exempt from further review research on existing data and records, that is, for data and records that have been collected previously and could be reanalyzed (see Box 2-1 for definitions, see also 45 CFR 46.101(b)(4)):

> (4) Research involving the collection or study of existing data, documents, records, pathological specimens, or diagnostic specimens, if these sources are publicly available or if the information is recorded by the investigator in such a manner that subjects cannot be identified, directly or through identifiers linked to the subjects.

---

[3]Some authors have turned more attention to the phrase "designed to" and concentrated on the initial intention of the investigators (see Amdur, in press). In HSR, however this criterion, while helpful, may still be ambiguous, since intentions may change as the project develops. As noted, projects that start as QA or QI may turn out to be publishable and then require IRB approval.

BOX 2-1 Terms for Less than Full IRB Review

The Common Rule codified in 45 CFR 46.101(a) states that except for those exemptions described in section (b), the policy applies to all research involving human subjects subject to federal regulation. The term "waiver" is sometimes used loosely, and may mean "federal guidelines do not apply," or "exempt from review," or "expedited review." If a project either does not meet the definition of research, or does not meet the definition of human subject involvement, then the Common Rule does not apply and the project is not subject to IRB review. This may sometimes be described as waiver of review, but in fact the project has been determined not subject to review.

Exempt—The Common Rule codified in 45 CFR 46.101(b) specifies that research activities may be exempt from the policy if human subjects involvement is limited to one of the listed scenarios, including studies involving the collection or study of existing data when those data either are publicly available or are not personally identifiable. As detailed in the text, however, some IRBs request to see the studies that may be exempt, and open files on them for tracking.

Expedite—The Common Rule codified in 45 CFR 46.110 specifies that research activities may be eligible for expedited review if the protocol involves only minimal risk or a previously reviewed protocol is receiving modifications that are only minor. Expedited review is carried out by the IRB Chair or by one or more experienced reviewers designated by the chair. Such expedited reviews have the force of full reviews, except that if the protocol is found not acceptable, then it must receive review by the full committee; the chair or designee alone cannot reject a proposal.

Waiver of Review—FDA regulations at 21 CFR 56.105 permit the agency to waive any of its requirements including the requirement of IRB review. Investigators would need to apply to the FDA for such a waiver. Since this report addresses HSR, not product safety and effectiveness, this provision is unlikely to apply (OPRR 1993, Chapter 2).

Waiver of Informed Consent—The Common Rule codified in 45 CFR 46.116(d) specifies that an IRB can alter or waive the requirement to obtain informed consent if it finds and documents that the research involves no more than minimal risk to the subjects, the waiver or alteration will not adversely affect the rights and welfare of the subjects, the research could not practicably be carried out without the waiver or alteration, and whenever appropriate, the subjects will be provided with additional pertinent information after participation.

Administrative Review—The terms "waiver," "expedite," and especially "exempt" were of concern to the committee because they may be misinterpreted by investigators, perhaps taken as indicating that the investigator

Continued

BOX 2-1 *Continued*

should determine whether a study needed IRB review. The committee proposes below and in Chapter 5 to substitute the term "administrative review" for all reviews that do not involve the full IRB. The committee was concerned that investigators may not understand how these terms are used in the federal regulations *and* may have a bias toward believing that their research does not require full IRB review. The committee recognizes, however, that others may have other suggestions for a new term. The committee's goal in this matter was to offer a term that recognized that some studies do not need full IRB review but does not seem to suggest that the investigator should decide what level of IRB review is needed.

Of course there are difficulties here too, in addition to those already discussed, such as the meaning of "recorded by the investigator." Some interpretations apply this exemption as long as no identifiers will be made public; others, if the investigator will not have the identifiers (although an assistant might); and others, only if no identifiers will be recorded by anyone. The OHRP has clarified that *information should be considered identifiable regardless of who holds the code that can link information to individuals, and the holder may be the researcher, the data provider organization, or some third party.* A particular problem in HSR that the regulations do not directly address is the possibility of identifying in databases individuals who have an unusual constellation of characteristics. Such indirect inferences can be made by using computer analyses and linking several databases. In addition, when the study participants are known to the investigators in other contexts, such as clinical care or community ties, the identity of individuals with rare characteristics can be inferred.

As the committee heard in the workshop, some institutions have an explicit policy requiring that all protocols be screened by the IRB, so that investigators are never placed in the position of deciding themselves whether their projects should be exempt from IRB review. The IRB or IRB office can ensure that the protocol meets the criteria for exemption from IRB review. Under this interpretation, the term "exempt" does not mean "exempt from any IRB oversight." Although the IRB may determine the protocol to be exempt from certain requirements, it may require others, such as periodic status reports. Often, the IRB chair and members who do the initial screening of potentially exempt protocols also carry out expedited review.

Some committee members suggested that the very term "exempt," although formally codified in the regulations, may be misleading. In particular, the regulations might mislead investigators to exempt their own research, when in fact the protocol may not meet regulatory criteria for exemption. In addition, some committee members remarked that the regulatory term expedited may be unfortunate, since surely both investigators and IRB members would wish all IRB reviews to be completed promptly. Finally, one possible solution might be to discard both terms in favor of "administrative review" since so many of these studies do receive quick turnaround review from the IRB chair and/or administrator.

What HSR May Qualify for Expedited Review?

The regulations also provide for expedited review of protocols in certain cases. An expedited review is carried out by the IRB chair or by one or more experienced IRB members. The DHHS publishes a list of categories of research that may be eligible for expedited review, including records research, which follows (63 FR 60364–60367, November 9, 1998):

> "(5) Research involving materials (data, documents, records, or specimens) that have been collected, or will be collected solely for nonresearch purposes (such as medical treatment or diagnosis)."

To qualify for expedited review, research must involve no more than minimal risk. The concept of "minimal risk" therefore plays a prominent role in determining whether a study qualifies for expedited review. Studies may not, however, qualify for expedited review if (63 FR 60364–60367, November 9, 1998)

> "[I]dentification of the subjects and/or their responses would reasonably place them at risk of criminal or civil liability or be damaging to the subjects' financial standing, employability, insurability, reputations, or be stigmatizing, unless reasonable and appropriate protections will be implemented so that risks related to invasions of privacy and breach of confidentiality are not greater than minimal."

If the reviewers do not approve the study for expedited review, it must receive a full IRB review.

May Informed Consent Be Waived?

For a project that *is* research involving human subjects and is *not* exempt, the IRB must ensure that the subjects have given free and informed consent to participate unless the informed consent requirement may be waived. In general, the IRB must ensure that the subjects receive adequate information about the research protocol, and its possible benefits and risks, in a form that is understandable to them; and that their consent was not coerced (45 CFR 46116(a)); and finally, that their consent was documented (45 CFR 46.117).

The requirement of informed consent may, however, be waived by the IRB if the research involves no more than minimal risk, the waiver will not harm the rights or welfare of the subjects, the research could not otherwise be practicably carried out, and when appropriate, the subjects will be provided with additional information after participating (45 CFR 46 116(d)). The concept of "minimal risk" is therefore a key element in determining whether informed consent can be waived.

What Is Minimal Risk?

Minimal risk, as defined in the regulations, "means that the probability and magnitude of harm or discomfort anticipated in the research are not greater in and of themselves that those ordinarily encountered in daily life or during the performance of routine physical or psychological examinations or tests" (45 CFR 46 102(i)). Like the terms discussed above, "minimal risk" can raise difficulties. For instance, it is not clear whether the terms "daily life" and "routine tests" refer to healthy people or to sick patients. In a clinical trial, the risk of side effects may be much greater in sick patients than in healthy volunteers. Other difficulties arise particularly in the case of HSR. On the one hand, in HSR projects that involve only analyses of previously collected data, there is no risk of physical harms such as an adverse reaction to an investigational drug or device. On the other hand, if a subject believes it reasonable to expect that medical records will not be disclosed for other purposes and the subject is later identified, he or she may well consider the risk to have been greater than ordinarily encountered and may feel wronged by a waiver of informed consent.

PREVIOUS STUDIES OF IRBs

Several recent studies have examined IRB function and procedures. The DHHS' National Institutes of Health (NIH) commissioned a large-scale study of IRBs that was released in May 1998 (Bell et al., 1998). This study concluded that the IRB system was functioning according to the regulations and was providing an adequate level of protection for human subjects although improvements were certainly possible. Many respondents to this study expressed concern about the large and rapidly expanding workload of IRBs. The following month, the DHHS Office of the Inspector General (OIG) released a study that highlighted several challenges to the IRB system (Brown (OIG), 1998b). This report noted that IRBs are facing greatly expanded workloads including new types of research. Furthermore, IRBs do not always have access to either the expert personnel or the training they would need in order to deal effectively with some of this research. The need for improved IRB training and access to expert consultants also arose in the present IOM study.

In February 1999, the U.S. General Accounting Office (GAO) released a report on IRB function in the specific context of medical records privacy (GAO, 1999). The GAO study observed that IRB review currently may not ensure the confidentiality of medical records when used in research. If the research is to be conducted at another institution, the IRB may rely on the confidentiality policies and procedures in place at that institution rather than carrying out its own assessment of the confidentiality of the data. Furthermore, the IRB may never even consider the issue of confidentiality if the study itself is eligible for exemption or expedited review according to the provisions of the federal regulations. Several of the respondents to the GAO study, however, detailed the information they require of investigators. These requirements, including statements of who will have access to the data and what provisions will protect the confidentiality of the data, were similar to some practices that were presented to the committee, which are highlighted in Chapter 3.

In April 2000, the OIG released an update reporting on conditions since its 1998 recommendations. According to the OIG, the problem of resources continues to plague IRBs. The OIG summarized its previous recommendation on resources and its current assessment:

> *"Prior Recommendations:* Require that IRBs have sufficient resources to adequately carry out their duties. Our recommendation was directed not only to staff and board member resources, but also to space, computers, and other essential elements. We urged OPRR (note: now OHRP) to hold institutions accountable for the resource commitments they made in their assurances.
>
> *Update:* OPRR's enforcement efforts have brought attention to IRB resource shortages at individual institutions and have led to additional support for IRB function at a number of those institutions—and quite likely at others that have taken note of the OPRR efforts. However, no further action has been taken to develop indicators of adequate resource levels or enable greater investments to support IRB functions. One approach that warrants more attention, and that NIH reports is under consideration, would be to allow an additional increment of grant funds to institutions to be used to provide necessary resources for IRBs. Such an approach could help reinforce to institutions and investigators that a well-supported IRB is a necessary cost of doing business. (Brown (OIG), 2000, p. 15)."

The IRB is the central feature of our human subjects protection system, so it is not surprising that the functioning of IRBs continues to generate great interest both in the federal government and in the nation generally. Subsequent chapters of this report suggest approaches that some IRBs have used with good success, but implementing them requires resources.

HUMAN SUBJECTS PROTECTION IN HSR

Within HSR, application of the three principles of human subjects protection (respect for persons, beneficence, and justice) to the subjects of data in large data bases becomes quite problematic, especially for researchers who may have no means of knowing the identity of the individuals. The general question of seeking informed consent poses a number of challenges, for example:

- In cases where large, rich databases already exist, a requirement to contact subjects prior to reanalyzing the data effectively would make it impossible to use the data for research (Iezzoni, 1999). All of the data would then be wasted, and no good research, hence none of the benefits of research, would be available.
- Further, the act of contacting the people requires more information and invades their lives, so if the information used in and resulting from the research did remain truly anonymous, the investigator would have violated the privacy of the

subjects anyway simply to tell them about an activity that might not be violating their privacy. Also, contacting individuals requires personal identifiers, so someone would have to know who was in the study, thereby raising the disclosure risk.

• Whatever the independent good of seeking informed consent in general, a requirement to seek it for HSR also could result in biased samples. The potential bias that would have to be considered could come about as described below.

    • Asking individually for consent to use data in a study lowers the participation rate. Asking people for permission to use their medical information in complex statistical models of health care systems may lead to increased confusion and unnecessary fear and anxiety. HSR can be difficult to explain to a nontechnical audience, and attempting to show why each variable is needed may give the audience the impression of being manipulated.

    • Because nonparticipants may differ from participants in significant ways, asking individually for consent will introduce bias that may not be possible to control.

    • As a result of bias from nonparticipation, the quality of the evidence resulting from the final analysis will be reduced.

    • Also as a result of bias from nonparticipation, the balance of benefit and risk in the study will be less favorable.

HSR investigators and their IRBs have concluded that individual informed consent, especially on a study-by-study basis, is one of the aspects of the clinical research model that is impossible to apply in research conducted by analyzing previously collected data. At the same time, the law presumably passed because a sizable number of citizens were concerned, which would be consistent with the results of a 1993 Harris Health Information Privacy Survey showing that 64 percent of respondents said their permission should be required before their records could be used in medical research, even if no personally identified information about them were published. In clinical research, specific informed consent is, as has been pointed out, the bedrock realization of the principle of respecting persons. In HSR, where the risks and the constraints are different, it is necessary to identify or develop alternative modes of respecting persons that will apply the principle in a feasible manner and address concerns about maintaining the confidentiality of the data.

PRINCIPLES AND PRACTICES

The application of the basic principles of human subjects protection in HSR raises specifically questions such as:

• how privacy ought to be protected,
• how confidentiality ought to be maintained, and
• how persons whose data are recorded ought to be respected.

Many responsible professional groups and expert individuals have developed sets of guiding principles for the treatment of health information.[4]

The objective of this study was to collect practices. Good practices should apply the principles of ethical human subjects research but also provide more specific guidance to investigators and IRBs than abstract principles can provide. In addition, good practices are flexible, taking into account the type of research and type of organization in question. That is to say, if we agree that we want to support HSR and obtain the benefits it has to offer, then we must identify and implement practices that adequately protect the subjects of HSR, while allowing worthwhile HSR to proceed. The committee hopes that the practices highlighted in the following chapters will facilitate HSR with appropriate and feasible mechanisms for the protection of human subjects, and will stimulate the development and dissemination of more advanced practices in the future.

The scope of this study, highlighting the empirical collection of practices, recognized that good normative principles are already codified in the federal regulations, but that no amount of codification can provide adequate direction for the day-by-day, study-by-study, work of an IRB. In short, regulations are important to provide norms, but they must still be implemented with the judgment and practical experience of individuals closest to the situation. This is what the local IRB system is designed to do. As apparent in Chapters 3 and 4, the sense of the committee is that the local IRB system is strong and the committee strongly supports HSR using it.

Any local IRB that reviews HSR will, however, have to understand the special problems of HSR and how to apply the federal regulations. The aim of sharing best practices is to support the local IRB with the good ideas already developed by other IRBs. One real challenge will be to find the best means of disseminating these good ideas (Chapter 5).

---

[4]Because different groups are developing principles to address different problems, or at least to address problems in different contexts, the sets of principles do not directly overlap in many instances—in particular, not mentioning a principle is not evidence that an organization would oppose it. These different perspectives make for difficult comparison (but see Buckovich et al., 1999). For example, several recommend removing personal identifiers as early, as and to the greatest extent, possible (GHPP, ISPE, Lowrance) or with some reservations (AAMC), many urge the proactive development of procedural and technical safeguards to protect privacy (GHPP, ISPE, JHITA, AAMC, Lowrance) and call for imposing penalties for breaches of confidentiality (GHPP, AAMC, JHITA, ISPE, PhRMA, Lowrance); some include specific protection for data access for research (AAMC, PhRMA); and several support the idea that individuals should be able to review their own records (GHPP, JHITA, ISPE, Lowrance).

3

Best Practices for IRB Review of Health Services Research Subject to Federal Regulations

Research with human beings is subject to federal regulations if it is federally supported or regulated for some other reason (e.g., will be submitted to the FDA as part of a new drug application). In addition, organizations that hold a multiple project assurance (MPA) from the Office of Human Research Protections (OHRP, formerly OPRR) usually, as a condition of the MPA, require all research at the institution to be subject to federal regulations, including research that is not federally supported. Furthermore, some organizations that do not hold such an MPA may also require all research to be conducted in accordance with federal regulations as a matter of organizational policy.

This chapter presents the recommendations and findings of the committee regarding the practices of institutional review board (IRB) review for health services research (HSR) that is done according to the federal regulations (whether the organization follows the federal regulations by requirement or by policy choice). The committee collected information from some universities and health centers and private research foundations, hearing testimony at a public workshop and collecting materials and statements from participating IRBs (see Appendixes A and B).

The committee was not able to conduct a comprehensive survey of IRB practices. The recommendations and findings that follow are based on the available data from a limited number of organizations and may not be representative of the entire IRB system. The committee presents these recommendations and findings in the hope that they may be helpful to some organizations, and may inform and stimulate further discussion about how IRBs can better fulfill their important role.

RECOMMENDATIONS

Recommendation 3-1. Organizations should work with their IRBs to develop specific guidance and examples on how to interpret key terms in the federal regulations pertinent to the use in HSR of data previously collected for other purposes. Such terms include *generalizable knowledge*, *identifiable information*, *minimal risk* and *privacy and confidentiality*. Organizations and their IRBs should then make such guidance and examples available to investigators submitting proposals for review.

The committee found that several topics cause considerable worry to investigators and IRBs because federal regulations are open to varying interpretations, with divergent implications.

The first of these topics is what activities are considered *research* and what criteria are used to operationalize the distinction between *research* and *other activities*. A key feature of the federal definition of research is whether the activity contributes to generalizable knowledge. In trying to distinguish research from activities such as quality assessment (QA) or quality improvement (QI) that use similar techniques to analyze personal health information in databases, however, both the federal regulations and the interpretations of these regulations by OHRP contain insufficient practical guidance for investigators and IRBs.

A second important issue is what constitutes *identifiable information* as defined in the federal regulations. Once again, the federal regulations provide little direction to investigators and IRBs on how to operationalize these terms, for example, whether or how it would be determined that data were *unidentifiable*, if they were coded in such as way that the investigator would have access to the data but also have great difficulty in reestablishing the identity of subjects.

A third issue is what constitutes *minimal risk* in HSR research and, in particular, what steps to protect the confidentiality of data in HSR suffice to allow the project to be considered as minimal risk. The issues of identifiable information and minimal risk have important implications for whether a project may be exempt from IRB review or receive expedited review or whether informed consent of research participants may be waived.

On all these issues, IRBs should communicate more directly with investigators and give local examples more specific than the guidance currently available in federal regulations and clarifications by OHRP. Clearer guidance would make IRB review more efficient as well as enhance the protection of subjects by helping to ensure that HSR projects incorporate confidentiality protections that the IRB finds important.

The committee found that IRBs vary in how they interpret federal guidelines pertaining to whether a project is intended to yield "generalizable knowledge" and thus should be subject to IRB review.

In the federal definition, research is "designed to develop or contribute to generalizable knowledge" (45 CFR 46.102(d)). The concept of generalizable knowledge seems to include both scientific rigor—to avoid error and to assure that findings can be widely applied—and an intent to disseminate the findings of the investigation. The IRB representatives participating in the workshop agreed that an activity would be considered research if the investigator plans to publish the findings. IRBs differ, however, in how they interpret other situations, particularly activities that might be considered QA or QI. Some organizations take an inclusive view of research, considering a project to be research if the findings will be disseminated outside the division or department that carried out the project. In this view, if the findings will be presented at a scientific meeting or to administrators from other organizations (e.g. other teaching hospitals), they will contribute to generalizable knowledge even if they are not published. Dr. James Kahn of the University of California in San Francisco, for instance, suggested at the workshop that if data are collected systematically, the project should be reviewed by the IRB, since it is reasonably likely that the investigator will publish the results if the findings are interesting (see Appendix B).

Ms. Angela Khan, IRB administrator from the University of Texas Health Sciences Center in San Antonio (UTHSCSA) explained at the workshop (see Appendix B) that her institution's IRB considers a number of issues in deciding whether a project is research rather than QA or QI. In assessing whether certain studies (generally only those directed toward internal QA) should be exempt from review, the IRB would consider whether

- the findings of the study will be disseminated beyond the department proposing to carry out the study;
- the protocol includes any change in clinical care or clinical processes that will affect other patients;
- the data to be collected would be available to the investigator only through the study (i.e., the investigator would not have access to such data in normal practice); and,
- there is any risk of harm or wrong to patients or staff.

If the answer to all of these questions is "no," then the UTHSCSA IRB would consider the protocol exempt as a QA activity. Other research may be exempt under the regulations but probably also would be reviewed at least by a subcommittee of the IRB, and informed consent might still be required. Ms. Khan also noted that generally the first consideration alone is sufficient to classify a project as research, since most investigators do in fact wish to publish their findings, even from projects that were planned as internal investigations, if they should prove interesting.

On the other hand, other IRBs use a narrower view of research. Dr. Robert Amdur of the University of Florida and also a presenter at the workshop (see Appendix B) suggested a contrasting approach. Starting from the premise that activities best characterized as QA or QI should be excluded from IRB review, he argued that publication (i.e., contributing to a lasting collection of generalizable knowledge), is a necessary condition for an activity to be considered research. Therefore if researchers say that they would *not* carry out the project if the results could *not* be made public, the project must be considered research. By contrast, for nonresearch activities such as QA or QI, there would still be sufficient internal organizational motivation for collecting the data, even though the activity would never increase the store of generalizable knowledge (Amdur et al., in press).

The committee found that another common dilemma occurs when the investigator does not initially intend to publish, and therefore does not ask for IRB review, but afterwards discovers the findings to be so interesting that they ought to be published. IRBs apparently vary in the way they handle such situations. Because the intentions of the investigators may change, other authors have suggested additional criteria for research, similar to those that some IRBs are already using. Casarett et al. (2000) suggest considering a QA or QI project as research if most of the subjects would not be expected to benefit directly from the knowledge generated and if the subjects would incur risks beyond those of normal practice.

The committee also heard that the determination of whether an activity is research, and hence how the observed individuals are to be protected, is particularly problematic in small organizations. Small organizations wishing to study their outcomes to improve their operations may not have access to resources for developing formal protocols and may not have an IRB that can review the project. Thus, an inclusive definition of research could preclude important projects in small organizations. In the workshop, participant Dr. Joanne Lynne of RAND gave the example of small hospices and home health care organizations who want to improve their own services but also share their findings with similar organizations, perhaps as part of a multisite study. The committee noted, however, that the likelihood of identifying individuals and the difficulty of maintaining confidentiality are both greatly increased in small organizations. Furthermore, in hospice care, information may be recorded about such sensitive topics as family disputes, emotional problems, or even illegal activities such as physician-assisted suicide. Hence individuals who are patients in small organizations and who are the subjects of projects carried out in small organizations that fall in the ambiguous zone between research and QA/QI, may be in need of the protection due human subjects; indeed they may be very vulnerable populations in need of strong protections.

The committee concluded that in light of these different viewpoints of various IRBs, investigators may be unclear how federal guidelines define research and how their own IRB will interpret those guidelines with regard to HSR.

The committee found that some IRBs have specific and detailed criteria for determining whether information is identifiable.

In the federal guidelines, research on existing data, documents, or records is exempt from IRB review "if the information is recorded by the investigator in such a manner that subjects cannot be identified, directly or through identifiers linked to the subjects" (45 CFR 46.101(b)(4)). Thus, the concept of identifiable information is crucial in determining whether an HSR project is exempt from IRB review. As mentioned in Chapter 1, the question of whether a record is identifiable is difficult because identifiability is not a property solely of the record itself but may be an inferential result of the record plus a linkage with some as-yet-unspecified database by an as-yet-undefined algorithm. How the question is answered has profound implications for the way the research in question will be regulated (Lo, 1999).

Ms. Khan noted that the UTHSCSA IRB, regarding projects using data from computer databases, asks the investigator to list all the fields to be collected and to indicate who will actually collect the data, how respect for confidentiality by any personnel involved will be ensured, and how further dissemination of the information will be prevented (e.g., storing data on computers that are not networked, storing codes identifying individuals separately from data, using passwords and/or key requirements to restrict access both to computers for data storage and to computer housing identifying codes). Another workshop presenter, Dr. Tora Bikson of RAND, suggested a general rule that RAND uses: if sorting data according to any variables produces subsets with ten or fewer members, these individuals will be at risk for identifiability by inference. The committee did not test or corroborate this cutoff point, which would require more theoretical work, but noted that rules of this type are good examples of useful practices.

The committee concluded that it is desirable for several reasons to have such explicit criteria on the identifiability of information. Explicit criteria improve the quality of HSR by promoting more careful consideration of the issue of whether information can be linked to identifiable individuals. Furthermore, explicit criteria promote consistency in the IRB review and allow more efficient review. If investigators know how the IRB determines whether information is identifiable, they can use that knowledge in study design to avoid problems such as building in unintentional identifiability. At the same time, it is important to remember that identifiability is a dynamic property, so it will never be possible to rely on a list of steps or an algorithm—the investigator and the IRB will have to think critically and exercise judgment in every case.

The committee found that IRBs vary in how they handle projects that may qualify as exempt from IRB review and in the formality of procedures for expedited review.

The committee heard that some organizations require any investigator to notify the IRB of all projects, including projects that might qualify for one of the exemptions in the federal regulations, and to submit annual status reports. By notifying the IRB of a project, the investigator would at least have the benefit of some external review of the protocol. Several organizations provide investigators with interactive on-line or at least printable forms that "walk" the investigator through a short deliberation about whether the protocol really qualifies for exemption from IRB review (see Box 3-1 and Figure 2 in Appendix B). On the other hand, other organizations allow investigators to decide for themselves whether a protocol is exempt from IRB review, and do not attempt to determine whether the investigator's decision is consistent with federal regulations. Still other organizations may allow the department head or chair to certify that a research project qualifies for exemption.

The sense of the committee is that any project benefits from at least some review from a party external to the project. In many projects, a review by an IRB chair or member alone may be sufficient, but even this quick review provides the project, the investigator, and most of all, the potential subjects with the benefit of an outside check that human subjects are adequately protected.

Likewise, clarifying the institutional procedures for expedited IRB review in HSR would have several salutary effects. It would call the attention of investigators to ethical issues regarding HSR. Furthermore, such clarification would encourage health services researchers to consider in a standardized way the issues of IRB review, patient consent, and protecting confidentiality. Clearer and more standardized procedures would make IRB operations more efficient, first, by allowing IRB members to focus their attention on difficult cases and, second, by giving investigators suggestions that IRBs currently request only after a protocol is reviewed, so that the investigators would be likely to submit proposals that incorporated these elements the first time. Finally, such standardization increases compliance with IRB policies and federal regulations that are intended to protect subjects in HSR.

Recommendation 3-2. IRBs should develop and disseminate principles, policies, and best practices for investigators regarding privacy and confidentiality issues in HSR that makes use of personal health data previously collected for other uses.

Confidentiality in handling health information is important for its own sake and for the enhancement of public trust in research. The committee heard several innovative and feasible ways to facilitate the maintenance of confidentiality.

The committee found that the identifiability of data in HSR is a continuum, such that absolute guarantees of confidentiality are impossible.

Even when investigators have made reasonable and good-faith efforts to de-identify data, to restrict access to a need-to-know basis, and to maintain confidentiality, the identity of an individual can sometimes still be inferred. The committee heard of examples in which individuals could be probabilistically identified from supposedly de-identified public use files. The committee also heard about the increased chances of identification within small populations (see

---

BOX 3-1 Excerpt from RAND's Human Subjects Research Screening Form

1. Will your project use either primary or secondary data collected from or about a living individual?
2. Are EXISTING DATA to be obtained or accessed, including official records, previously collected survey data, or other extant information? (specify as many as apply:

- Anonymous unrestricted public use data.
- Anonymous but restricted use data.
- De-identified private data (neither RAND nor a primary contractor or subcontractor for the research [if any] can link data to individuals, although a third party [e.g., an HMO, a government agency, a school district, or other data provider] may be able to do so).
- Identifiable data (data that can, in principle, be linked to individuals by RAND or by a primary contractor or subcontractor for the research [if any], either through direct identifiers or arbitrary code numbers associated with direct identifiers).
- Other:

[Additional questions address types of interactions with subjects and types of interventions.]

NOTE: See also Figure 2 in Appendix B.

Appendix B). These probabilistic identifications by inference result from unforeseen links between the de-identified data in one database and complete or identifiable data from another source. It is also, of course, always possible for a human employee mistakenly to allow data to become available.

Many health services researchers and IRBs have developed practical and specific procedures for protecting privacy and confidentiality in HSR projects that involve analyses of previously compiled databases. For example, researchers in health services may need to identify individual subjects to combine data from different datasets or to compare follow-up information with baseline data. Such projects can still protect subjects by using computer-generated identifiers or by encrypting the data, rather than identifying individuals by name, hospital record number, or Social Security number. When the project requires definite linking, the researcher will have to use unique individual identifiers, such as Social Security number, Medicare Health Insurance Claim number, health record number, or some unique code generated within the project for this purpose, to establish that records in different datasets belong to the same person. However, relying on a single linking variable can lead to some errors if the number is entered incorrectly for a particular transaction (hospital stay, doctor's office visit). Therefore, prudent investigators would, if possible, use some other attribute as a corroborating linking variable, such as sex or date of birth. Probabilistic linking, in contrast, reflects the fact that people can share identifying attributes such as names and birthdates, so that investigator is not certain that the linked records belong to the same person.

In other cases the identifying information needed for accurate data merging may not be specific to the patient. For instance, a study on hospital characteristics might require the names of hospitals to merge Medicare Part A claims files with the American Hospital Association survey database, but would not have to identify specific patients. In addition, researchers can take additional steps to prevent the identification of individuals with unusual characteristics (see also Table 3-1 for further detail). There may be only a few individuals of a given age with a rare diagnosis in a certain zip code who were hospitalized between certain dates, and such individuals may be readily identified by inference because there are so few persons with these characteristics. Researchers can, however, change the recording of the data so that there are more records in each data cell. For instance, it is harder to identify individuals if the investigator records the year of birth rather than the exact birthdate, the first three digits of the zip code rather than the entire zip code, and the number of hospitalized days rather than the exact dates of hospitalization. Furthermore, researchers can reduce the number of outliers on a scale by collapsing categories at the extremes of the scale. For instance, the researcher can set the highest value for a cost-of-hospitalization data field at something greater than a certain dollar amount, rather than retaining the exact figures for high-cost hospitalizations. Although there can be no absolute guarantees of confidentiality, these measures reduce the likelihood that individual subjects would be identified. If adopted more widely where appropriate, these procedures would enhance protections for subjects of HSR. At the same time, it is important for IRBs to bear in mind that different techniques are appropriate in different research projects, so different subsets of these techniques might be applicable or not usable in different studies.

The committee found that IRBs were able to suggest many ways in which protocols could better protect confidentiality with simple measures.

The committee heard of cases that illustrated problems or potential problems with confidentiality that IRBs had averted. In some studies, investigators planned to record identifiers with the data even though there was no need to maintain the identifiers. In fact when the IRB questioned the necessity for using identified data, the investigators realized they simply had never thought of whether their research required the identification and they immediately removed them. In another instance, already mentioned, that was reported to the committee at the workshop, one participant described finding his own HIV results projected in a meeting with personally identifying information, with no other purpose than showing an example of records in the database. In both cases, the basic problem appeared to be that the persons collecting data had not considered the confidentiality implications of their methods. These examples demonstrate the usefulness of a review independent of those involved in the protocol.

The committee also found that some IRBs give detailed attention and clear advice to investigators on how better to protect confidentiality at various steps of an HSR project.

Ms. Khan said that for any protocol involving particularly sensitive data, the UTHSCSA IRB requires the investigator to obtain a federal certificate of confidentiality. The certificate of confidentiality is a legal mechanism (described in the Public Health Service Act, Section 301(d)) designed to protect certain types of sensitive data from subpoena (see Wolf and Lo, 1999). The committee also heard, however, from organizations that store such sensitive data in facilities outside the United States to protect them from discovery processes (the committee did not, however, seek legal opinions as to whether such a strategy would provide effective legal protection from discovery). Colonel Anderson, IRB chair at the United States Army Medical Research Institute of Infectious Disease, reported that the Army's procedures specify that that an investigator may request that research records be maintained on request under special coded identification numbers, with a linkage to the individual's Social Security number. The key linking the study identification number and the Social Security number is then stored separately under extremely limited access. In general, networked, distributed, and backed-up digital information and environments together pose new types of threats to privacy. Some researchers, for instance, may not realize that taking a diskette with backup files home to work on a personal computer that is connected to a DSL line (that is on all the time) creates a serious security breach. Such examples suggest that the role of technical experts may yet be underappreciated.

The committee found that violations of privacy and confidentiality might occur in HSR studies that have small numbers of subjects in cells, but that careful IRB review including appropriate consultation with persons knowledgeable about any specific community norms may help investigators to revise protocols to reduce such risks.

The committee heard that small, isolated minority communities and their individual members might be particularly vulnerable to breaches in confidentiality, often unintended. The risk is increased in situations where the number of individuals is small and the individuals are readily recognized by others in the community. If a project targets a particular rural county or Indian Reservation, for instance, there may be only one or a few individuals with a particular characteristic (e.g., giving birth to twins) and these individuals would be readily identified in the local situation even if their identity were effectively hidden from strangers.

At the same time, the risk of loss of the confidentiality veil and exposure to stigma is increased for the individuals and for the community as a whole if the community is relatively small and its members are readily recognized as members by the majority society. It would be important for those IRBs that review such research to consider concern for the community as a whole, but might be effected through protection of individual members, since U.S. legal tradition contemplates privacy as belonging to individuals, not groups. For example, a study designed to assess the need for certain health services can at the same time have the effect of identifying the community with a negatively valued characteristic (such as underuse of prenatal care or, more strongly, drug or alcohol abuse during pregnancy as evidenced by neonatal symptoms). In this case, all members of the community where the need has been shown may suffer stigma even if not involved in the study or not possessing the characteristic in question.

The risk may be increased still further by the presence of culturally significant identifiers that are not recognized as sensitive private information by researchers who are not familiar with the community and therefore do not mask all the sensitive data fields. For example, specific locations, occupations, or other characteristics may indicate a very small subgroup even within a minority community (e.g., a few members of a particular tribe on a reservation inhabited primarily by another tribe), so that those individuals could be unintentionally identified. Similarly, among some Native Americans, revealing the name of a particular lodge or other immediate grouping could be considered an invasion of privacy.

Dr. Freeman of the Indian Health Service IRB pointed out that many such mistakes could be avoided by consulting with the community for unanticipated risks to privacy (see Appendix B). For example, the name of the lodge need not be disclosed in a publication; the site of the study might be identified simply as a tribe in a certain state. Dr. Freeman also noted that a minority community may be particularly apt to worry about mistreatment from researchers, and any perceived mistreatment at the hands of one researcher will have negative impact on the ability of future researchers to gain community cooperation. Members of the committee also noted that there may be no generally agreed-upon spokesperson to represent the community, but even if there are multiple overlapping groups involved, the IRB could ensure that the investigator had consulted several representatives and at least had some input even if it is not possible to have a definitive or comprehensive statement.

The committee found that the particular issues of the use of minors as subjects are connected mainly with informed consent and assent by the subjects. Specific cases in which children are at elevated risk, however, such as when they have been removed from their parents due to domestic violence, demand additional care and protection for these vulnerable subjects.

The committee found that when children are the subjects of HSR that makes secondary use of previously collected data, there are situations in which the risks of breach of confidentiality may go beyond the risks existing for adult subjects. In such situations, investigators and IRBs should take special care to ensure that these vulnerable subjects are protected. In the type of HSR addressed in this study, including analysis of data collected for some other purpose, informed consent for each study is generally not practicable and the challenge for researchers is to build in appropriate confidentiality protections so that the risk to subjects will truly be minimal. As discussed in Appendix C, "minors" is not a homogeneous class, and the potential for psychosocial risks such as embarassment vary with age within the class. In many cases, the when risk of confidentiality breach in general has been minimized effectively, the committee sees no greater risk to minors, in respect of their being minors, than to any other subject. In specific cases, such as perhaps research on domestic violence and foster care, individual children might be identifiable because they are in a relatively small group. Furthermore, if subjects are identified, they may be at risk for being removed from a parent or guardian even though better placement options may not be available. Thus, the confidentiality of these subjects' identity should receive extra scrutiny. It is also true that records research might reveal patterns of injury, perhaps allowing abuse of a child to be detected and stopped. The committee also found that certain variables, such as hospitalizations, are so much rarer among minors than among older adults that special consideration for protecting the confidentiality of these variables as potential identifiers is warranted. As with the previous finding regarding subjects who are members of small minority communities, protecting the confidentiality of data on minors will be enhanced by an IRB whose members or consultants are knowledgeable about the particular issues of a study and about the relevant developmental changes of the minor subjects involved, and can help highlight variables of unusual identifying potential.

Recommendation 3-3. IRBs should redesign applications and forms (paper and electronic) tailored to HSR that analyzes data originally collected for other purposes and then distribute them widely (e.g., post them on-line) to assist investigators in writing the human subjects sections of their HSR proposals and in preparing applications for IRB review. IRBs should be knowledgeable about the differences between HSR and clinical research, and any forms developed should reflect these differences.

A checklist or logical series of questions lays out the criteria that the institution has adopted to determine, for example, what constitutes research. These instruments are useful in several ways: they call the attention of investigators to ethical issues arising in HSR, and they help investigators to think through systematically the specific issues regarding IRB review, patient consent, and protection of confidentiality.

Interactive forms and checklists can make IRB review more effective and efficient. Investigators can see if their projects might meet criteria for waiver of informed consent, expedited review, or exemption from review. If necessary, the investigators can revise their study without the delays involved in resubmitting a revised hard copy of the protocol to the IRB and waiting for review by the IRB staff or a board member. Such forms would allow IRBs to focus their review, again by drawing attention to difficult cases. Overall, interactive forms would enhance compliance with IRB policies and federal regulations and would make review less burdensome for investigators and IRB members alike.

The committee found that some organizations make use of interactive on-line forms to help investigators determine whether a project should be considered research and whether it qualifies for expedited review.

In general the committee was favorably impressed with organizations such as RAND that had devised interactive on-line forms to minimize investigator time and paperwork requirements.

RAND has implemented an on-line system to help ensure that there is appropriate IRB review of all protocols. The brief on-line questionnaire in Box 3-1 initially helps the investigator determine whether the project might require IRB review. If the questionnaire so indicates, then a more detailed questionnaire helps the investigator explore the alternatives of exemption from IRB review, expedited review, or full review see (Figure 2, Appendix B). The on-line system may indicate that a project would not fall into the category of full IRB review if it uses only anonymous or public use datasets, or de-identified datasets if neither RAND nor any another party on the contract has access to the identifiers. In addition, the IRB is notified whenever a project receives an internal funding account number—in fact, assigning such a number automatically triggers a message to the investigator to start the questionnaire. The system is designed to be inclusive, that is, to send any borderline cases to IRB members for specific attention. In more difficult situations, the IRB chair and/or selected members would have to decide whether the particular project could be exempt. Examples of situations in which an IRB members would have to become involved to decide whether further IRB review might be needed include projects that will use anonymous or nonsensitive primary data gathered through surveys, interviews, or other methods requiring a direct interaction with subjects; projects that gather data from public officials or candidates; or intervention research that is anonymous and without risk.

The committee did not hear of comparable automation in a university setting but found that automating the burden of paperwork as much as possible would increase compliance and reduce burdens on both investigators and IRBs. Just as increased protections come at the price of increased investment in equipment and expertise, so would it be necessary for organizations to invest in IRB operations improvements to increase their efficiency.

As has been mentioned, the committee concluded that, principal investigators intending to involve human subjects should not be in the position of exempting themselves—with or without forms and guidance documents; rather, the protocol should receive at least some outside review. At the same time, forms such as those by RAND would be helpful in facilitating prompt and high-quality review. The design and dissemination help the institution, the IRB, and the investigator systematically approach questions such as whether an activity is research. In another example, a university-based IRB showed how the university was working to help its investigators ascertain whether projects would be classified as research or QA and/or QI. There, the investigator is asked to consider whether the proposed study contains any of the following elements, which the institution has recognized as potentially associated with research rather than QA or QI:

Characteristics of projects using HSR methods that are research, not QA or QI:

- Exploring any previously unknown phenomena
- Collecting information beyond that routinely collected for the patient care in question
- Comparing alternative treatments, interventions, or processes
- Manipulating a current process

To which might be added:

- Being intended for publication if possible

Although the committee would wish the IRB chair or designee to corroborate an investigator's assessment of a project as rather than research, the preparation of systematic materials such as the above list would facilitate review.

Recommendation 3-4. IRBs should have expertise available (either on the committee or through consultants) to evaluate the risks to confidentiality and security in HSR involving data previously collected for some other purpose, including the risks of identification of individuals and the physical and electronic security of data.

The committee urges IRBs and investigators to consult information technology and data security experts about protecting confidentiality in their specific situations. It is not the intent, nor would it be possible, for this committee or this report to provide an adequate basis for a data security program.

The committee found that the IRBs would probably benefit from guidance on how confidentiality can be protected so that IRB members have more background on what to look for in a protocol.

The committee followed the lead of previous IOM and National Research Council (NRC) reports regarding the question of how to protect confidentiality and considered protecting access to the data per se, as well as protecting individual subjects by manipulating the data after they have been collected.

BOX 3-2 Summary of Technical Protections for Sensitive Data

Individual authentication of users. To establish individual accountability, every individual in an organization should have a *unique* identifier (or log-on ID) for use in logging onto the organization's information systems. Strict procedures should be established for issuing and revoking identifiers. Where appropriate, computer workstations should be programmed to automatically log off if left idle for a specified period of time.

Access controls. Procedures should be in place for ensuring that users can access and retrieve only that information that they have a legitimate need to know.

Audit trails. Organizations should maintain in retrievable and usable form audit trails that log all accesses to clinical information. The logs should include the date and time of access, the information or record accessed, and the user ID under which access occurred. Organizations that provide health care to their own employees should enable employees to conduct audits of accesses to their own health records. Organizations should establish procedures for reviewing audit logs to detect inappropriate accesses.

Physical security and disaster recovery. Organizations should limit unauthorized physical access to computer systems, displays, networks, and medical records; they should plan for providing basic system functions and ensuring access to medical records in the event of an emergency (whether a natural disaster or a computer failure); they should store backup data in safe places or in encrypted form.

Protection of remote access points. Organizations with centralized Internet connections should install a firewall that provides strong, centralized security and allows outside access to only those systems critical to outside users. Organizations with multiple access points should consider other forms of protection to protect the host machines that allow external connections. Organizations should also require a secure authentication process for remote and mobile users such as those using home computers. Organizations that do not implement either of these approaches should allow remote access only over dedicated lines.

Protection of external electronic communications. Organizations should encrypt *all* patient-identifiable information before transmitting it over public networks, such as the Internet. Organizations that do not meet this requirement either should refrain from transmitting information electronically outside the organization or should do so only over secure dedicated lines. Policies should be in place to discourage the inclusion of patient identifiable information in unencrypted e-mail.

Software discipline. Organizations should exercise and enforce discipline over user software. At a minimum, they should install virus-checking programs on all servers and limit the ability of users to download or install their own software. These technical practices should be supplemented with organizational procedures and educational campaigns to provide further protection against malicious software and to raise users' awareness of the problem.

System assessment. Organizations should formally assess the security and vulnerabilities of their information systems on an ongoing basis. For example, they should run existing "hacker scripts" and password "crackers" against their systems on a monthly basis.

SOURCE: Excerpted from NRC,1997; pp. 8–9, Box ES.1.

Protections based on controlling access to sensitive data include procedural disciplines, such as making data available only under licensure agreements and training personnel not to use methods such as fax or Internet transmission that are not secure means of transferring data. Other ways of protecting data from unauthorized access include technical means, such as installing software that requires user authentication, and physical protections, such as guarding laptops with sensitive data while traveling and storing sensitive data where it would be safe from access (which may include storage outside the country for protection from subpoena, although the committee did not ascertain the reliability of this strategy).

Previous reports from the National Academies have discussed technical means of protecting data privacy and maintaining confidentiality. *For the Record* (NRC, 1997); included a detailed list of technical and organizational measures for immediate adoption (see pp. 8–9, Box ES.1) to enhance confidentiality protection. The technical protections are shown in Box 3-2.

The feasibility of these measures was demonstrated in a proof-of-concept project at a large medical center (Halamka et al., 1997) by a team including a member of the earlier NRC committee (Peter Szolovits, also a member of this committee). The committee emphasizes that this report is not the place to recommend a detailed data security program but suggests that IRBs consider the protective measures already described and implement them if they have not done so. The committee also emphasizes that increased protection comes at an increased cost, which requires investment, generally in both equipment and expertise, by the organizations conducting research.

Protections based on manipulating the form of the data after collection have also received detailed examination in previous NRC reports. *Private Lives and Public Policies* (NRC, 1993) addressed the confidentiality and accessibility of government-held statistics generally and recommended confidentiality measures including data-masking techniques such as topcoding (setting an upper limit on a range of values [e.g., age 70 and over], so as to avoid reporting increasingly rare outlying values in ranges where they would be isolated—see Box 3-3 for other examples). Many of these measures are also feasible for handling data in general, not only government-held databases. As with any manipulation, however, each technique has disadvantages as well as advantages, so the committee emphasizes that it is important for the investigator to have flexibility in applying the techniques best suited to the particular research question and dataset(s) of the protocol.

Again, the committee emphasizes that this study could not undertake detailed presentation of data-masking techniques, but suggests that investigators and IRBs consider the protective measures already described and implement them where possible if they have not done so. Ideally, these technical and data-masking safeguards for confidentiality would be implemented in the context of policies and procedures adopted by the organization for all uses of personal health information, including clinical care, business activities, or research. The chair of the *Private Lives and Public Policies* committee (George Duncan, also of a member of this committee) noted that many government agencies including the Bureau of the Census and the National Center for Health Statistics have significant experience with the release of data with confidentiality protections and should be consulted in future work.

This committee notes that it may also be helpful for investigators and IRBs to have access to specific lists of potential direct identifiers for removal. Such lists of procedures and specific identifiers may, however, never be exhaustive and, as stated in the previous finding, a set of guaranteed conditions may not be possible.*

The committee found that some organizations provide IRBs and investigators access to experts in information technology.

RAND has installed a three-person privacy team as part of its IRB. The team includes an information resource specialist (who specializes in security measures such as encryption and creating codes to substitute for identifying data), a data librarian (who specializes in rules and practices for dealing with large datasets acquired from other organizations), and a networks specialist (who specializes in conditions and limitations of safe data transfer over the network). These professionals help design and implement data-safeguarding plans commensurate with the level of risk for various protocols. The committee concluded that in light of rapid developments in information technology (IT), such access to expertise in information technology is highly desirable.

Most IRBs do not, however, have the power or resources to implement data security programs on their own, and their time must be devoted to reviewing research proposals, protocols, and annual reports. What IRBs can do is reject studies that do not have acceptable data security measures, while at the same time working to understand the value of reductions in the incidence and severity of security breaks relative to the cost of increased security precautions. The host

---

*As an example of a good beginning of a list for identifiers to be wary of, the committee referred to 164.506(d)(2)(ii)(A) of the proposed rule (DHHS, 1999). The list includes name; address; names of relatives or employers; birth date; telephone, fax number, or email address; medical record; health plan beneficiary, account, certificate/license number; vehicle or other device serial numbers; Web universal resource locator; Internet protocol address number; voice or fingerprints; photographs; or any other unique identifying number characteristic or code that the covered entity has reason to believe may be available to an anticipated recipient of the information. The confidentiality of data that were de-identified to this extent would be better protected, but as noted, the data might still allow the probabilistic identification of persons by inference with other data sources. The proposed rule accounts for this possibility with an additional condition stipulating that if data are to be disclosed, then the covered entity must have no reason to believe that any anticipated recipient of such information could use the information, alone or in combination with other information, to identify an individual. As has been noted, however, this condition may be impossible to satisfy.

organization and research sites are usually the loci of data security programs. These organizations determine their own level of investment in IT and levels of affordable data security. The committee therefore concluded that IRBs should obtain consulting services from data security experts to gain better understanding of the expected yield in reduction of the likelihood of break-ins to a secured data system produced by alternative security programs.

Recommendation 3-5. Institutions that carry out HSR and train health services researchers should require that trainees, investigators, and IRB members receive education, with updates as technology changes, regarding the protection of privacy and confidentiality when using data previously collected for another use.

Education is critical not only for IRB members, but also for researchers, technicians, and any other employees who may come in contact with health information. Better education about how to protect confidentiality and possible sources of risk will help investigators design better confidentiality protection into their proposed studies from the start. Better education of all employees who may come in contact with the data will help raise the level of understanding and alertness throughout the organization.

The committee found that organizations vary in how they educate IRB members about research ethics and federal guidelines. The committee found that learning on the job may be inadequate preparation for IRB members.

The committee heard at the workshop that some IRBs have apparently not had the opportunity to gain experience with HSR and may ask for incongruous changes. Some organizations provide training for IRB members in formal courses or seminars, or by providing orientation materials (OPRR, 1993). Several organizations send members to professional meetings and seminars, such as those sponsored by the organization Public Responsibility in Medicine and Research (PRIM&R). Certainly informal education from more experienced IRB members and administrators provides continuing training during IRB meetings. As noted earlier, the OIG has already observed that IRBs are facing greatly expanded workloads, including new types of research, and do not always have access to either the expert personnel or the training they would need in order to deal effectively with some of this research. At the same time, IRBs often face serious resource limitations, which in turn affect training.

The question of the OHRP's role in IRB member education was raised at the workshop, not only disseminating regulations as the office currently does, but also the possibility of OHRP's collecting and disseminating information about the best practices of IRBs. Dr. Puglisi, representing OHRP, said that information and guidance are posted on the OHRP website, and that the OHRP is actively expanding its educational activities.

BOX 3-3 Sample "Restricted Data" Tools for Providing Data While Protecting Confidentiality

Tool	Advantages	Disadvantages
De-identification—Removing personal identifiers such as names, addresses, telephone numbers, e-mail addresses, Social Security number	Clearly necessary so that a person is not immediately linked to a record	Data may still be at risk of disclosure. A data snooper may be able to re-identify a record—uncover the identity of a record—by linking certain key variables in the record to those in some separate and complete identified record held by the snooper. For data analysis, this makes it impossible to add additional variables or to guarantee for future retrieval the ability to contact individuals about adverse findings
Coarsening—Releasing the data in categories or broadening the size of categories. Includes top-coding and bottomcoding—creating categories at the extremes of the data	Makes re-identification more difficult since several subjects may have the same values in the records	Decreases the information content of the data and makes certain statistical techniques, such as regression, more difficult to apply
Dropping unnecessary variables	Makes re-identification more difficult because there are fewer key variables present for linkage and because fewer records are unique in their values	Dropped variables may later prove useful in analysis of the data
Dropping records that are easy to identify, usually with unusual combinations of values	Lowers disclosure risk	These records may be of particular interest to a researcher.
Geocoding—replacing person-specific information with the average from a geopolitical unit in which the person resides	Makes re-identification more difficult	Decreases information about unusual persons in the geopolitical unit. The geopolitical unit may be inappropriate for a specific research project
Aggregating units to a higher-level group—(e.g., providing average values for all patients with the same health care provider)	Values released do not correspond to a particular individual	Loss of information when the within-group variability is nonnegligible

BOX 3-3 *Continued*

Tool	Advantages	Disadvantages
Random error injection(e.g., adding independent zero mean random perturbations to each data value)	Makes record linkage through key variables more difficult.	Loss of information, also can make data analysis more complicated
Winsorizing(e.g., removing highest values, replacing with the mean of values removed)	Preserves mean of group, hides unique upper values	Loss of information, especially on upper-value cases

The committee found that some organizations require training of investigators in research ethics and IRB procedure.

Many investigators in HSR are initially trained in a variety of disciplines, including clinical medicine, pharmacy, epidemiology, and health administration, but rarely specific programs in HSR. Training investigators as well as IRB members may greatly enhance human subjects protection and speed the initiation of good research. Educational activities must, however, be designed to target the needs and time constraints of adult learners who are also busy researchers. In particular, training should be tailored to the type of research methods that researchers use—the ideal training for clinical trials investigators would not be helpful for health services researchers. Several organizations require, or are planning to require that investigators pass a course on human subjects protection before their protocols can be reviewed. NIH already requires that intramural investigators pass an on-line course on research ethics and regulations. The committee believes such education should be encouraged and expanded, provided that this is feasible for the already heavy schedule of most investigators. The committee heard some promising ideas about how to provide this training, such as on-line tutorials, but several members noted that there could be resistance at some institutions to making any training a requirement, because of the heavy workload that many investigators already carry.

In addition to formal courses, IRBs play an important role in educating investigators through individual discussions regarding specific projects. IRB administrators and chairs participating in the workshop reported that their organizations function more effectively as collaborative educators than when trying to function as enforcers and that collaboration also effectively reduces the need for enforcement.

Recommendation 3-6. Health care or other organizations that disclose or use personally identifiable health information for any purpose including research or other activities using HSR methods should have comprehensive policies, procedures and other struc-

tures to protect the confidentiality of health information and should have in place appropriate strong and enforceable sanctions against breaches of health information confidentiality.

Access to specific expertise and enhanced general education are important, but the committee also observed that the human element of the research enterprise necessarily includes human potential for error and even malfeasance. Therefore organizations should complement and support the proactive strategies of expertise and education for better confidentiality protection with deterrents to wrongdoing. Such sanctions ought to be graded according to the offense (e.g., whether the incident was a simple mistake or an intentional violation) and should apply not only to researchers but to all employees of the organization.

4

Best Practices for IRB or Other Review Board Oversight of Health Services Research Not Necessarily Subject to Federal Regulations

This chapter presents the recommendations and findings of the committee regarding the practices of organizations conducting research or quality assessment or quality improvement activities that are not necessarily subject to federal regulations. The committee collected information from health care provider organizations (Intermountain Health Care and HealthPartners), a pharmacy benefit management company (Express Scripts), and the epidemiology section of a pharmaceutical company (Merck). The committee heard testimony at a public workshop and collected materials and statements from these organizations (Appendixes A and B).

As in the previous chapter, the reader should note that the committee was not able to conduct a comprehensive survey of private organizations that utilize health information, much less to collect all their practices for maintaining confidentiality. The recommendations and findings that follow are based on information from various organizations, but neither the committee nor the informants make any claim to be representative of the entire segment of the industry. The committee presents these recommendations and findings in the hope that they may be helpful to some organizations and may inform and stimulate further work in this area. The committee believes that studies involving human subjects should be reviewed similarly whether the study is subject to Common Rule provisions or not. As a result, the committee has recommendations in this chapter that are similar to those in the Chapter 3. The committee decided to keep two separate chapters in part because the implications of the recommendations might be different for different types of organizations, and also because the separate structure seemed to reflect the committee's charge more clearly.

The committee was impressed with the commitment to privacy and confidentiality that the representatives of several private companies presented at the workshop. Companies appear to be at different stages of developing internal privacy or confidentiality policies regarding HSR and should be encouraged to continue to develop these organizational policies and procedures. The committee believes this recommendation to be consistent with the spirit of proposed federal regulations on privacy (DHHS, 1999). It is, however, outside the scope of this project to make a detailed critique of those regulations.

RECOMMENDATIONS

Recommendation 4-1. Researchers should have all HSR reviewed by an IRB or other review board regardless of the source of support or whether the research is subject to pertinent federal regulations.

Recommendation 4-2. IRBs and other boards that review HSR that is not subject to federal regulation should assess their practices in comparison with the best practices of IRBs working under pertinent federal regulations and, when the latter offer improvements, adopt them. Alternatively, when their own practices are superior though not subject to federal regulation, they should share them with IRBs applying the Common Rule.

IRBs, or other suitable review bodies, offer a review of research projects by knowledgeable persons not directly associated with the project. This independent review protects subjects of research because independent reviewers may identify concerns and suggest ways to minimize risks that were not apparent to investigators. The committee heard several examples of protocols that were or could have been substantially improved with respect to confidentiality by relatively simple modifications. Research subjects, who undergo risks for the benefit of science and society as a whole, should have the protections of such independent review as a matter of ethical best practice, regardless of funding source. There is little ethical justification for making a distinction between the level of protection afforded subjects in federally funded projects and that given subjects in projects funded by private sources if the risks to these subjects are comparable; indeed, proprietary projects could have additional conflict-of-interest pressures and thus might greatly benefit from outside review.

The committee found that some organizations and their IRBs apply the federal regulations to all health services research, regardless of funding source even though they are not legally required to do so.

The committee commends this consistent approach and notes that well-designed review operations, procedures, and practices, some of which are highlighted in the previous chapter, should allow the extension of IRB or other review board oversight without creating significant additional burdens for researchers or review boards. In addition, this would allow both researchers and potential subjects to benefit from a review that is independent of the study staff, for instance, by identifying potential investigator–subject communication problems early on.

The committee believes that the best practices identified in the previous chapter are feasible to implement in electronic data systems, provided that the institution has the resources to do so and that implementing them can substantially increase confidentiality. In general, the techniques mentioned are "practices" precisely because they are already in use at some institution (see also Halamka et al., 1997). These practices include using codes, rather than identifiers such as Social Security numbers or names, to locate a record and a variety of measures to reduce the likelihood that individuals can be identified by inference.

In particular, the committee recommends the following observations from the previous chapter to institutions that do HSR and similar work that is not subject to federal regulations.

As in Recommendation 3-2, IRBs or other review boards should develop lists of principles, policies, and best practices on protecting privacy and confidentiality in HSR for use by investigators. Because the identifiability of data in HSR is a continuum, so that absolute guarantees of confidentiality are impossible, it is critical to take all reasonable steps that can synergistically enhance confidentiality, such as the areas of consideration listed in Boxes 3-2 and 3-3.

As noted in Recommendation 3-3, the committee suggests that the development and on-line posting of applications and review forms specifically designed for HSR would improve the quality of review of HSR projects. IRBs and other review boards in any setting should be educated about the differences between HSR and clinical research, and any forms developed should reflect these differences.

As mentioned in Recommendation 3-4, IRBs or other review boards should have available expertise (either on the committee or through consultants) to evaluate the risks to confidentiality and security in HSR, including the risks of identification of individuals and the physical security of data. The committee urges review boards and investigators in any setting to consult information technology experts about protecting confidentiality in their specific situations. It is not the intent of, nor would it be possible for, this committee or this report to provide an adequate basis for a data security program.

Also, as stated in Recommendation 3-5, organizations should require that researchers and other employees who come in contact with confidential health information receive education in the handling of this information to maintain confidentiality.

The committee concluded that principal investigators intending to involve human subjects in research or for other types of investigations should not be in the position of exempting themselves; rather, the protocol should receive at least some outside review. Such a check by knowledgeable, independent individuals will facilitate consistently high standards of treatment for all confidential health information in research and for all subjects whose data are so used.

> **Recommendation 4-3. Health care organizations that conduct projects applying the methods of HSR to personally identifiable health information for purposes such as QA or QI, disease management, and core business functions as well as for research should have comprehensive policies, procedures, and other structures to protect privacy when personal health information is used for research or other purposes.**

Intermountain Health Care, a large, integrated health care organization, reported that most violations of confidentiality occurred outside the research arena, in areas such as clinical care and business activities. This distribution is not surprising, because most uses of personal health information are in these nonresearch areas. From the viewpoint of the patient, it does not matter whether a violation of confidentiality occurs in a research project or other activity because the risks of being harmed or wronged may be the same. Publicity about violations or alleged violations of confidentiality undermines public confidence in both health care operations and research.

The committee found that companies that purchase, deliver, and/or reimburse health care services could likely engage in many activities that analyze personal health information using the same techniques as HSR, which fall into the "gray zone" between research and nonresearch described in the workshop summary (see Figure 3 in Appendix B).

As detailed in the earlier report *For the Record* (NRC, 1997, see especially, pp. 66–68, Table 3.3), health care organizations use personal health information for clinical care, billing, payment, quality improvement, and business planning. The need to make personal health information accessible for these purposes must be balanced with the need to respect the confidentiality of such information.

The committee found that some organizations have developed comprehensive policies and procedures regarding the confidentiality of personal health information that are best practices. These comprehensive policies apply to research as well as to other activities making use of personally identifiable data.

A comprehensive program has several facets: organizational components such as a privacy board that recommends and implements policies; procedural components including an active training and enforcement program for all employees, technical components such as the use of audit trails to detect unauthorized uses of personal health information; and a suitable board to review research projects. Comprehensive organizational privacy policies and procedures apply to researchers as well as clinicians and administrative staff. A review board can be more certain that confidentiality is protected in research if the organization has a strong, comprehensive policy.

The committee heard that Intermountain Health Care (IHC) has an Information Security Committee that may be similar to the privacy boards described in the proposed rule. The IHC Information Security Committee (IISC) is constituted similarly to an IRB, including community members, as well as line administrators, researchers, and computer specialists. The IISC works closely with the IRB on activities on the HSR side of the continuum. The IISC is also responsible for determining whether projects from the ambiguous area in the middle of the health care operations/research spectrum should proceed to seek IRB review. Finally, the IISC generates and recommends data security policies to the Board of Trustees of the company and then helps implement these policies and procedures throughout the organization, thus enhancing confidentiality protections at the operations end of the continuum.

Recommendation 4-4. Health care or other organizations that disclose or use personally identifiable health information for any purpose including QA or QI, disease management, and core business functions as well as for research should have in place appropriate, strong, and enforceable sanctions against breaches of the confidentiality of health information.

Committee members agreed that previous experience provides ample evidence that, although most investigators and staff are upstanding, there will always be a few who are subject to the temptation to misuse access to confidential information. In fact, the committee felt that this aspect of human subjects protection may have been neglected and therefore recommends consideration of deterrent policies for organizations working with IRBs under the Common Rule and for the organizations considered here. Such individuals and, even more, the subjects of any research projects that they may come in contact with, would benefit from a credible threat of sanctions for improper use or inspection of confidential information. Such sanctions ought to be graded according to the offense, (e.g., whether the incident was a simple mistake or an intentional violation) and should apply not only to researchers but to all employees of the organization. Just as in organizations that have IRBs, it is important that the proactive approaches of expertise and education toward proper handling of confidential information also be complemented and supported with sanctions against mishandling information.

The committee heard at the workshop that at the personnel level, all IHC employees must sign a confidentiality agreement, which must be renewed every two years, and then comply with a "need-to-know" policy limiting who has access to which data. The company also tracks data access with automatic elec-

BOX 4-1 Summary of Protections for Sensitive Data

Organizational Practices

Security and confidentiality policies. Organizations should develop explicit and clear security and confidentiality policies that express their dedication to protecting health information. These policies should clearly state the types of information considered confidential, the people authorized to release the information, the procedures that must be followed in making a release, and the types of people who are authorized to receive information.

Security and confidentiality committees. Organizations should establish formal points of responsibility (standing committees for large organizations, a single person or a small committee for small organizations) to develop and revise policies and procedures for protecting patient privacy and for ensuring the security of information systems.

Information security officers. Organizations should identify an information security officer who is authorized to implement and monitor compliance with security policies and practices. The security officer should maintain contact with relevant national information security organizations.

Education and training programs. Organizations should establish programs to ensure that all users of information systems receive some minimum level of training in relevant security practices and knowledge regarding existing confidentiality policies *before* being granted access to any information systems.

Sanctions. Organizations should develop a clear set of sanctions for violations of confidentiality and security policies that are applied uniformly and consistently to all violators, regardless of job title. Organizations should adopt a zero-tolerance policy to ensure that no violation goes unpunished.

Improved authorization forms. Health care organizations should develop authorization forms that will improve patients' understanding of health data flows and limit the time period for which authorizations are valid. The forms should list the types of organizations to which identifiable or unidentifiable information is commonly released.

Patient access to audit logs. Health care providers should give patients the right to request audits of all accesses to their electronic medical records and to review such logs.

SOURCE: NRC, 1997. Page 9, Box ES.1.

tronic logs and has designed the electronic records system to ensure that identifiable portions are accessible only to designated employees. IHC terminates employment because of privacy infractions.

Many of the provisions in Recommendations 4-3 and 4-4 are consistent with the recommendations regarding organizational practices discussed in *For the Record* (NRC, 1997) and quoted in Box 4-1. As noted in Chapter 3, the committee emphasizes that a complete analysis of organizational structures and processes to enhance the maintenance of confidentiality is beyond the scope of this project but recommends that organizations consider these practices and implement them as appropriate, if they have not already done so.

The committee encourages health care organizations to adopt provisions that are practicable in their circumstances. Comprehensive policies for all uses of personal health information will avoid issues of how to oversee activities that are in the gray zone between research and QA or QI. If a comprehensive policy is in place, a QA or QI project will have strong confidentiality safeguards that make the risk to patients minimal.

5

Recommendations for Next Steps

"The end of this study will not be the end of studying [the issue of privacy and confidentiality in health services research]," said Dr. Michael Fitzmaurice of the Department of Health and Human Services' (DHHS') Agency for Healthcare Research and Quality (AHRQ), one of the agencies sponsoring this study, during the committee's workshop. The committee endeavored to stay strictly within the focused charge for the project. In the course of the study, however, the committee identified many important issues in addition to institutional review board (IRB) practices that should be addressed if subjects of health services research (HSR) are to be protected adequately. Throughout this report the committee has tried to refer inclusively to IRBs and/or other review boards (unless circumstances specified only IRBs). The term "IRB" has regulatory implications of the extension of federal oversight in a new area. The term "privacy board" has been used in a rule that, as this report was being written, had been proposed but not finalized and may mean different things to different people.

The committee has also tried to emphasize that any HSR should be reviewed according to the ethical principles reflected in the federal regulations and further that the reviewers should be knowledgeable about HSR and privacy protection and should be independent of the research group. Although not all HSR is in fact subject to federal regulations, the committee concluded that the review of HSR ought to follow the principles of these regulations.

RECOMMENDATIONS

Recommendation 5-1. Institutions whose IRBs or other review boards review HSR should ensure adequate administrative support and funding for review bodies and should incorporate improving review operations into overall institutional strategic planning, and organizations that sponsor HSR should also support designating adequate funds for such review.

The committee corroborated previous reports that questioned whether IRBs have the resources to carry out their mission. The committee noted especially the April 2000 update report of the DHHS Office of the Inspector General, (OIG). This report, *Protecting Human Research Subjects: Status of Recommendations*, concluded that the resource problems identified in the OIG's 1998 report, *Institutional Review Boards: A Time for Reform*, still exist. The committee heard that many IRBs already have a heavy workload of proposals for review and that most members serve in a voluntary capacity. Additional resources will be required to implement the best practices described in Chapters 3 and 4.

The committee found that IRBs (or any other review boards) need adequate funding specifically to review HSR.

As just mentioned, previous reports have documented the need for adequate funding of IRBs. The committee heard corroborating evidence that resources continue to be a problem for IRBs. A recent committee at the University of California at San Francisco, an institution conducting a great deal of research involving human subjects, recommended that high priority be given to adequate IRB staff support, increased use of computerized information systems, and increased funding for training investigators about IRB function (see also Appendix B).

In addition to adequate resources for staff and committee members, IRBs or other review boards need additional funding for new activities that could make their work more effective and efficient. With regard to HSR, for example, review committees need access to more expertise in information technology, such as how investigators can reduce the likelihood that subjects will be identified through the use of coding and encryption and through defining variables in ways that eliminate data cells having a small number of subjects with an unusual set of characteristics. Furthermore, human subjects protection programs will require additional resources to put into place the kinds of computer decision support systems that would enhance the effectiveness and efficiency of reviews of HSR studies and better ensure that these studies have in place appropriate safeguards for confidentiality.

The committee also heard a number of proposals for how to provide the resources that human subjects protection committees would need to carry out their missions adequately. Dr. James Kahn, IRB chair at the University of California in San Francisco, proposed that IRB review be added as a line item in grants, doubting that sufficient overhead funds would be directed to IRB support at a large university that has many other competing uses of overhead funds (this proposal is very similar to that suggested in the 1998b and 2000 OIG reports). Some committee members argued that support of the IRB, manifestly a necessary overhead cost of supporting a human subjects research program, is a particularly appropriate use of overhead funds. In fact, Dr. Kahn reported that UCSF had commissioned an ad hoc committee to review the UCSF IRB's function. The ad hoc committee was asked to consider the composition, procedures, and support of the IRB and whether it could be of better service to the university. The committee returned a list of recommendations, including several suggestions about increasing the use of electronic information systems, as well as increased training for researchers to address both research responsibilities and institutional procedures, and increasing staff support for the human subjects protection program. In addition, Dr. Kahn specifically suggested designating 1 to 1.5 percent of each grant using human subjects to be earmarked as funding for the human subjects protection program. Independent IRBs, of course, charge investigators or institutions a set fee to review protocols.

Determining the resource needs of IRBs and analyzing how to provide the necessary support in different organizational contexts, although far beyond the scope of this report, are important issues that must be addressed. Groups such as the American Association of Medical Colleges (AAMC), Public Responsibility in Medicine and Research (PRIM&R), and Applied Research Ethics National Association (ARENA) can play key roles in addressing these issues. Particular attention has to be given to how to support innovative uses of computer technology that would make IRB review less burdensome and help train investigators in research ethics and IRB requirements.

Recommendation 5-2. The DHHS and other federal departments and private organizations such as the Association of American Medical Colleges (AAMC), the Association for Health Services Research (AHSR, but now known as the Academy for Health Services Research and Health Policy), the American College of Epidemiology (ACE), the International Society for Pharmacoepidemiology (ISPE), Public Responsibility in Medicine and Research (PRIM&R), the Applied Research Ethics National Association (ARENA), and others should continue or expand educational efforts regarding the protection of the confidentiality of personally identifiable health information in research.

While these recommendations highlight DHHS as the sponsor of this study and a major sponsor of relevant research, the recommendations should be applied by other Common Rule signatory departments and agencies as well. The committee believes that the approach of identifying best practices for IRB oversight of HSR is a fruitful one that should be further developed. Recommendations of best practices will provide more specific guidance to investigators and

IRB members than is currently available. This approach draws its strength from the commitment of both IRB members and administrators and of researchers to protecting the rights and welfare of the subjects of HSR. Both IRBs and scientists have developed useful practices that, if more widely adopted, could lead to improved protection of confidentiality and privacy, without creating undue burdens. Private organizations can play a crucial role in developing and publicizing best practices. Professional societies such as AHSR, ACE, and ISPE are composed of investigators who carry out studies analyzing large databases of data previously collected for other uses. AAMC represents medical schools that train researchers and carry out a great deal of HSR. PRIM&R and ARENA members review HSR studies and help educate investigators about the protection of human subjects. All of these organizations can help identify and disseminate best practices for the protections of privacy and confidentiality in HSR. Ultimately, such best practices for data security or confidentiality protection should be developed for each of the other specific types of data collection methods used in HSR including, but not limited to, focus groups, mail surveys, telephone surveys, personal interviews, home visits, interactive data collection via the Web, and remote sensing, as well as secondary analysis of health data that have already been collected for some other purpose.

The committee found enthusiasm and openness to new ideas on the part of the IRBs and investigators who participated.

The committee was impressed that in the spirit of scientific collaboration and competition, many health services researchers, IRB members, and IRB administrators were receptive to good ideas and wanted to excel in how they protect confidentiality in HSR. As with any other aspect of research, there is a great deal to be gained when people from different institutions exchange ideas and experiences. These stakeholders recognize that public confidence that personally identifiable health information will be used appropriately is crucial to the continued ability to carry out important HSR projects in a timely fashion. The committee found that these stakeholders were dedicated to resolving the tension between confidentiality and access to personally identifiable health information for HSR in an ethically acceptable manner.

The committee observed that the general willingness of IRB administrators, chairs, investigators, and organizations whose research is not subject to federal regulations to participate in its workshop and to consider and try ideas that had been developed at other institutions indicates that the distribution of information on best practices would likely be well received. Such recommendations should be transmitted to investigators and IRBs through the Internet, as well as through presentations at professional society meetings and workshops, and in training grants and awards, program grants, and center grants.[1] This committee, because of the time frame, could take only the first steps in identifying best practices for IRB review of HSR. Further efforts, including more systematic input from IRBs and health services researchers, could lead to more specific and comprehensive suggestions for institutions and investigators to adopt.

The difficulty in the dissemination of information about best practices identified through this approach may be in locating a central venue and keeping it up to date. The DHHS can promote interactions among scientists and IRBs that will lead to wider dissemination of good ideas regarding the oversight of HSR and protection of the subjects of HSR. Through its roles in funding HSR, supporting training programs in HSR, and overseeing human subjects protection, the DHHS can have great impact on strengthening IRB review of HSR while allowing valuable research to proceed. In the long run, greater public confidence that personally identifiable health information is adequately safeguarded will promote more support for HSR and perhaps avoid the restrictive legislation and regulation that some European nations have adopted (see for example Appendix D).

The committee found that identifying best practices is a promising approach to strengthen the protection of HSR, while allowing valuable studies to proceed in a timely and practical manner.

The committee found that the federal regulations and the interpretations and guidance issued by OHRP do not provide sufficiently specific guidance for many issues regarding HSR. As discussed earlier in this report, IRBs and investigators admit that they struggle with such difficult concepts as identifiable information and the definition of HSR. Bringing together people who grapple with these issues is likely to lead to greater agreement and clarity.

Based on these findings, the committee believes that DHHS should convene meetings that will facilitate these exchanges of ideas and identify feasible best practices that institutions might choose to adopt more widely. The meetings should include health services researchers, IRB members and administrators, leaders of institutions that carry out HSR, experts in information technology, experts in ethics and law, and public representatives. Such interdisciplinary expertise will be needed to resolve the complex problems regarding the protection of subjects of HSR. The working group should draw on the expertise of organizations that are required to handle sensitive computerized personal information in a confidential manner. Such organizations would include commercial firms transacting business over the Internet as well as government agencies such as the Bureau of the Census and the National Center for Health Statistics. Although the committee was unable to consult with these organizations because of time con-

---

[1] Informal communication already flourishes through the Medical College of Wisconsin IRB (MCWIRB) list serve (see www.mcwirb.org) and should be encouraged and enhanced however possible.

straints, it recognizes that such expertise would be extremely useful to health services researchers.

In addition, the committee identified from material presented at the workshop several topics that require additional discussion. These include how to contact persons identified through secondary data analysis using large databases for more intensive interviews in those instances where it is possible and necessary to identify and contact subjects (often neither is true of HSR); how to review multisite HSR projects, particularly those carried out in small health care organizations that do not have IRBs; and how to ensure that HSR projects involving children take into account the changing needs, vulnerabilities, and capacities of children as they mature (see, for example, Appendix C).

Recommendation 5-3. Organizations that furnish health services researchers with personally identifiable health information should ensure that the data are prepared in a manner that protects confidentiality adequately.

The committee heard several instances reported at the workshop where HSR investigators requested de-identified data from federal agencies but received data that had not been de-identified because the agency in question lacked the resources to do so.

As large holders of personally identifiable data, the situation of federal agencies having to choose between providing data that have not been de-identified, or simply refusing to provide data for research at all, is worrisome. Organizations holding health data should develop and/or implement lists of points to consider in reviewing data requests with respect to protecting privacy and confidentiality in HSR.

Similarly, either such holders of information should require that the health services researcher submit evidence that the proposed research has undergone IRB review, or the data holder should review the study through its own independent review process.

Committee members observed further that if data suppliers possessed more highly developed data warehouses so that investigators could always go back to the source to pick up forgotten variable(s), health services researchers would be more likely to ask for only those variables they really believe they will need. When data requests are limited to a one-time, take-what-you-need process, investigators are prone to ask for much more than they expect to need just in case they might be forgetting something.

Recommendation 5-4. The funders of HSR should be willing to cover the cost of preparing personally identifiable health information that is collected in clinical care, billing, or payment so that confidentiality can be adequately protected in HSR.

The committee found that health services researchers and other data handlers need sufficient funding to protect adequately the confidentiality of personally identifiable health information.

The committee heard examples of how health services researchers lacked the resources to adopt computer-based measures that would strengthen confidentiality in important HSR. For example, a health services researcher at a leading academic hospital reported that she was finding it increasingly difficult to obtain consultation from their excellent medical informatics group because these experts were over-committed to other projects.

The committee concluded that adequate resources to consult with and pay for the services of computer experts will be essential if confidentiality is to be adequately protected in HSR. In most cases, funders of HSR will have to allow such computer consultation and services as line items in grants. The need for such support should be accepted as an integral cost of high-quality HSR.

Recommendation 5-5. The DHHS should continue and expand efforts to encourage holders of personally identifiable health information to make this information available to researchers as public use files after suitable application of techniques to minimize the risks of identifiability.

If an organization holding health data has made a dataset publicly available without restriction, as is done with the National Health Interview Survey (NHIS), then projects using only such data can be considered minimal risk and eligible for exemption per 45 CFR 46.101(b)(5). In order to promote HSR, data-holding organizations should consider making as much data available in the public domain as is safely possible. The committee notes that the Interagency Confidentiality and Data Access Group has developed a checklist for use in considering whether data may be released, which helps holders of data develop such public use files.[2] This group is affiliated with the Federal Committee on Statistical Methodology, an interagency committee first convened in 1975 and dedicated to improving the quality of Federal statistics.

Recommendation 5-6. The AHRQ should consider supporting a feasibility study on developing procedures for facilitating linkage of separate data files containing sensitive data from different sources to create analytical files such that it would be possible for researchers to create linkages that are reliable and informative, and at the same time, to protect the confidentiality of the original data disclosure through de-identification and other protective measures so as to save

---

[2]Confidentiality and Data Access Committee, Federal Committee on Statistical Methodology. Checklist on Disclosure Potential of Proposed Data Releases (July 1999): http://www.fcsm.gov/spwptbco.html.

the subject from being placed at risk of harm or wrong through improper re-identification.

Much of the value of retrospective, database-oriented research comes from the ability to draw inferences from data derived from different sources. The committee urges interested parties including DHHS agencies to encourage research on linkage and anonymization with a view toward two goals: first, to create linkages that are reliable and informative, and second, to approach as closely as possible the goal of anonymized data.

The ability to link records to one another may be very important, though that does not mean that the data need to be linked to the identity of the individual. Health care organizations may have to identify episodes of illness in a patient, which may be found in records of emergency room visits, ambulance services, hospital stays, operative records, bills from independent medical providers, rehabilitation services, pharmacies and pharmacy benefit managers, and so forth. To recognize that the data drawn from these various sources refer to the same individual, it is important that researchers be able to identify the same patient in each set of records. This identification allows joining of these various datasets into a single (logical) database that contains all relevant data about the patient. Such identification and joining is often difficult and is one of the motivations for keeping names or other direct identifiers in the records. The true identity of any given individual is not really necessary to merge databases; all that is required is some unique identifier, such as a code, which could be difficult to re-associate with the actual patient. Ideally, then, the various sources of data would have their records indexed by the same set of identifiers, but ones that are not easily re-associated with the actual patient's identity.

There are several possible ways to address this problem. One suggestion exploits developing cryptographic and authentication technology to create health information identification systems (as explored in a pilot study of Kohane et al., 1998, described in greater detail in Box 5-1). Such a system would have the advantage of allowing different databases to be linked through an identifier that could be certified as associating records about the same individual but would be difficult for any user to decode. As different projects were designed, the investigators could specify different types of health identifiers to maximize values in various dimensions including the extent to which the identifying code could be used in other projects and the degree of security surrounding it. Since the program designed by Kohane and colleagues generates identification systems (not a particular identification code), the resulting flexibility and complexity of the identifiers would be much less vulnerable to decoding than a single certified identifier such as a Social Security number, while still allowing database linkage.

BOX 5-1   Sample Tool for Creating Health Information Identification Systems

The Tool: A computer program called the Health Information Identification and De-Identification Toolkit, or "HIIDIT" (pronounced "hide it")

What HIIDIT does: Health identification systems allow the creation and use of identifiers to refer to particular individuals, institutions, IRB's, studies, etc. HIIDIT supports the designer of a health identification system to select appropriate properties of such a system, such as whether the identifiers are global in scope or unique only within a specific institution, whether a single centralized directory of identifiers is kept or if such directories are held only locally for small groups of individuals, whether the identifiers are associated with individuals by a recognized national authority or more local means such as a notary public, and whether the identifiers are publicly known or limited to use by specific groups. Based on a choice among such design criteria and on a carefully defined set of operating rules specific to the design, it is usually possible to select a set of technologies that implement a health identification system meeting the criteria.

As an example, consider a possible design of an identification system for a regional genomic database, in which a number of different *source sites* (clinics) contribute genomic data to a *study site*, where each source site and the study site also have IRB's. The study is to operate under the following rules: (1) Only duly authorized data are entered from any source site into the study. (2) Although the identity of the patient is known at the source site, it should be very difficult to determine from data at the study site. (3) The study data should only be accessible with permission of the study site's IRB. (4) A source site should be able to add data to a patient's record in the study without giving away the identity of the patient to the study. (5) If the study's IRB approves, the study site can contact the source site's IRB, who can in turn identify the patient so that the source site may contact the patient for additional information, but all without revealing the identity of the patient to the study site.

In this example, HIIDIT uses the methods of *public key cryptography* to generate cryptographic key pairs for each patient, each source site, the study site, and each IRB. Within each pair, the *public* key is known to everyone, but the private key is known only to the patient or responsible individual(s) at that site or IRB. Each key in a pair is the inverse of the other. According to well-known public key principles, this permits, for example, a source site to *encrypt* a message with the study site's public key. Only the study site can then successfully decrypt this message by using its secret private key; thus, the message is secure against prying eyes in transit. Similarly, a source site can *sign* a message by encrypting it with its own private key, after which any recipient can verify that the message must have come from that site by successfully decrypting it with that source site's public key. These techniques are often used in combination to send messages that are unreadable and unalterable by anyone other than the sender and receiver. In the example, the source site computes the identifier under which a patient's data will be stored at the study site by the following steps:

BOX 5-1 *Continued*

1. Sign the patient's public key with the source site's private key. Call the result the *source id.*
2. Encrypt the source id with the source IRB's public key.
3. Append the result of step 2 and the source site's public key, then encrypt the result with the study site IRB's public key. This result is the *study id* for that patient.

The Result: One may verify that the design rules are enforced by the implemented technique. For example, it is possible to verify that the study site's IRB can determine from which study site a particular patient's record arose, but cannot identify the patient. That source site's IRB can, in turn, identify the patient if it chooses to use its own private key. A properly designed set of rules and a correct implementation can assure that data are successfully shared, but without likely risk to the patient's privacy.

How HIIDIT could fail: Identification systems designed using HIIDIT are most vulnerable to unauthorized disclosures in the same way that any other system for protecting confidentiality is vulnerable, namely, if the information professionals at an institution are careless (or unscrupulous) when they input data so that they either gain unauthorized information or permit others access to it. HIIDIT can shift the level of security along the health information privacy spectrum toward greater anonymity, but it cannot replace the need to provide staff with rigorous and comprehensive training and policies.

SOURCE: Kohane, Isaac S.; Dong, Hongmei; and Szolovits, Peter. Health Information Identification and De-Identification Toolkit. *Proceedings of the American Medical Informatics Association* Symposium 1998: 356–360.

Another type of linkage system would depend on trusted third parties to be responsible for linking the separate data files. These entities could hold the keys linking individuals to the data. After merging datasets, this entity would then strip off the identifiers, check that identification cannot be (reasonably) inferred[3], and take any needed steps to protect the data. This approach has the advantage of being simpler to implement, specifically because it requires that many fewer organizations and individuals develop high degrees of technical competence and organizational commitment to use standard procedures. The disadvantages are related to the centralization of the linkage operation.

The committee notes that the question of how precisely to perform the data file linkage in any particular case is not straightforward but varies depending on the characteristics of the specific research question and data used. At the same time, such merges can be technically complex, so access to a central, highly

---

[3]The committee recognizes that the question of how difficult identifiability by inference must be in order to make data safe for release will continue to be a matter of debate and notes that the standard should be expected to change as technology changes.

skilled facility to perform them could improve the overall efficiency of the research enterprise. There is, however, an additional theoretical risk that such trusted entities, because they are known to hold large amounts of personally identifiable health information, may be the target of intruders. Thus there is a need to test the feasibility of this approach, regarding both the capability of a central facility to be flexible with the technical needs of different types of projects and the safety of a central merging facility.

Recommendation 5-7. DHHS (AHRQ and/or NIH) and other federal departments or agencies should consider developing and supporting a research agenda concerning IRB protection of subjects from nonphysical harms such as risks to privacy and confidentiality in human subjects research (including cultural meanings of privacy and confidentiality).

Such a research agenda would likely include current IRB practice, as well as new procedures and policies to provide better human subjects protection, and also would include monitoring of IRB practices. A systematic study of nonphysical risk assessment was beyond the charge given to this committee, and the committee would in any case have found itself unable to accomplish it due to limitations of time and in respect of the Office of Management and Budget (OMB) rules on extensive surveys. The committee found, however, that such information would be of great use both as a baseline and, if updated periodically, as a basis of continuous policy evaluation. The findings would be of use to IRBs, researchers, regulators, and any other parties interested in privacy and confidentiality.

Recommendation 5-8. The OHRP should review the possibility of proposing a change to the regulations with respect to HSR to replace the terms "exempt" and "expedite" with "administrative review."

The committee is recommending this review only with respect to HSR—the committee did not investigate possible consequences for other types of research that might be affected if the change were applied to all research on human subjects. The committee heard several reports that well-intentioned and conscientious researchers may judge a study to be exempt from review under the current regulatory language and therefore never bring it to the attention of a review board. Since the committee has concluded that all HSR should receive some review by a board that is independent of the research project, the committee suggests that this possibly misleading terminology be avoided. The committee recognizes, however, that a change to the Common Rule involves coordination among many agencies and may therefore be difficult to achieve. The committee further recognizes that others may have other suggestions for a new term. The committee's goal in this matter was to offer a term that recognized that some studies do not need full IRB review but did not seem to suggest that the investigator should decide what level of IRB review is needed.

Recommendation 5-9. Health services researchers, and institutions that participate in and benefit from HSR, should voluntarily adopt best practices for IRB review of HSR.

The committee found that some policies intended to strengthen confidentiality and privacy may have serious adverse consequences for HSR.

The committee found that some nations have adopted laws or regulations that allow individuals to exclude their personally identifiable health information from databases, that require written consent from patients for use of health records for research, and that require the anonymization of data for any secondary data analysis. Such measures were enacted to protect the confidentiality of computerized personally identifiable health information (see Appendix D).

The committee learned, however, that some measures intended to promote privacy and confidentiality may have serious adverse consequences for HSR (AAMC, 2000; AHSR, 2000). A requirement of individual informed consent would render impossible valuable HSR, notably projects using HMO, insurer, or Medicare and Medicaid databases. Furthermore, population-based studies would be biased if people could exclude themselves from research. Even if studies were possible, their results could be misleading because persons who agree to HSR may be different in important and unpredictable ways from persons who refuse to participate. In addition, a requirement that all secondary data analyses use only anonymized data would make it impossible to conduct valuable HSR that requires follow-up of a cohort or the linking of data from different datasets. Thus, some measures intended to strengthen privacy and confidentiality may lead to invalid studies and be a poor basis for public policy decisions.

If patients and members of the public in general do not find that they can trust that confidential information will be protected throughout research, they may seek further measures to protect confidentiality. Some such measures could be detrimental to HSR. The committee therefore urges investigators, data users and data holders and publishers to voluntarily adopt and continually upgrade the best practices of IRBs and other review boards in ensuring the protection of data privacy and confidentiality in HSR.

Recommendation 5-10. All stakeholders in HSR should support strategies to improve the protection of privacy and confidentiality without impeding research.

The committee found it necessary to encourage further study beyond the scope of its charge. Although there was not time in this project to explore wider-ranging ideas, the committee suggests several as potential starting points in a multifaceted strategy to improve the awareness of privacy issues and improve confidentiality protection practices:

- DHHS could sponsor a conference to include health services researchers, journal editors and editorial boards to discuss inclusion of privacy protection methods in journal articles and requiring evidence of IRB review as a condition for publication, and HSR-related journals and health care management journals could sponsor special issues devoted to health data privacy and confidentiality and could refuse to publish results from studies that had not received IRB review.
- DHHS should investigate revising the Public Health Service grant application guidelines to incorporate a formal section on data privacy or confidentiality protection in the human subjects section of the application.
- DHHS could include data privacy experts on scientific peer review panels that are charged with the review of HSR proposals.
- Funders of HSR, including DHHS, HMOs, and private companies and foundations (perhaps working through a professional organization such as the AHSR), should consider issuing a special research solicitation on data protection methods, to include research on methods of attacking security protections.
- PRIMR and organizations supporting HSR could sponsor a conference on the equitable selection of subjects for research. Certain populations may be over-solicited as subjects of current HSR projects, because of availablity of suitable databases, federal requirements to have minorities adequately represented, or policy interest in certain topics, such as the impact of poor access to health care. Questions for consideration could include whether participation in many studies may increase the risk that confidentiality will be breached and harms or wrongs occur as a result, and, whether there may be a risk of stigma if a group is overrepresented in current research, even if individual subjects who are members of the groups are at minimal risk for having their individual confidentiality violated.
- Universities and colleges should conduct special one-week courses in data security for students majoring in HSR and related fields.
- Organizations with special interest in data privacy and good-quality HSR should consider sponsoring a prize competition, perhaps annually, for the best privacy and confidentiality practices by a health care organization. This might be akin to the Malcolm Baldridge National Quality Award, which has had such an impact on quality assurance in industry. Given the importance currently being placed on privacy and the attendant competitive value that an organization may see in winning such an award, there may well be sufficient incentives for organizations to put forth their best ideas and document them in a way that is understandable. Such a prize competition could be seen as a positive side of such awards as the Annual UK "Big Brother" Awards, which highlight egregious

breeches of privacy,[4] but would really be more like the Malcolm Baldridge award in spirit, with health data privacy protection as the focus.

The methods of HSR, applied to data previously collected for other purposes, have been useful in discovering and demonstrating systemic effects and population-level trends in the organization and delivery of health services. It is important that we, as a society, continue to have access to such research in order to inform policy making in both private and governmental arenas. At the same time, it is important that we, as a society, protect the privacy of individuals and of vulnerable groups, and the confidentiality of information that patients share with health care providers. As a result of the present study, the committee has concluded that it is possible both to carry out valuable HSR and to protect confidentiality. However, to do so will require adequate funding. Resources are needed to support dedicated, trained IRB members and staff, to establish organizational confidentiality policies and electronic security practices, to educate researchers, and to provide statistical and computer expertise. The true test of our commitment to the twin values of advancing useful knowledge and protecting confidentiality is whether we are willing to make the needed investments to achieve both goals.

---

[4]For the Malcolm Baldridge National Quality Award, see http://www.quality.nist.gov. For the Big Brother Awards, see http://www.bigbrotherawards.org/. Note that the organization also recognizes achievements in privacy protection, but generally within the United Kingdom.

References

Amdur, Robert, Speers, Marjorie A., and Bankert, Elizabeth. IRB Triage of Projects that Involve Medical Record Review. In press.

Applebaum, Paul S. Threats to the Confidentiality of Medical Records—No Place to Hide. JAMA. 2000 Feb 9; 283(6):795–796.

Association of American Medical Colleges. AAMC Comments on The Recommendations of the Secretary of Health and Human Services on the "Confidentiality of Individually Identifiable Health Information." AAMC Testimony Presented to the Senate Labor and Human Resources Committee. 1997 Nov 10.

Association for Health Services Research. Definitions of Health Services Research. 2000.

James Bell Associates. Review Draft—Final Report Evaluation of NIH Implementation of Section 491 of the Public Health Service Act, Mandating a Program of Protection of Research Subjects (NO1-OD-2-2109). 1998 May 19.

Belmont 1979. The Belmont Report. Office of the Secretary. Ethical Principles and Guidelines for the Protection of Human Subjects of Research. The National Commission for the Protection of Human Subjects of Biomedical and Behavioral Research. 1979 April.

Bradburn, Norman M. Population—Based Survey Research. Presentation Done at National Bioethics Advisory Commission. 2000 Apr 6.

Brainard, Jeffrey. An Inside Look at How a University Tries to Protect Human Subjects. The Chronicle of Higher Education. 2000 Mar 17:A31.

Brooks, John M.; Doucette, William, and Sorofman, Bernard. Factors Affecting Bargaining Outcomes Between Pharmacies and Insurers. Health Service Research Selected Papers From The Association for Health Services Research Annual Meeting, June 21–23, 1998. 1999 Apr; 34(1 Part II):439–451.

Brown, June Gibbs, Inspector General. Institutional Review Boards: The Emergence of Independent Boards. Department of Health and Human Services, Office of Inspector General. 1998a Jun.

Brown, June Gibbs, Inspector General. Institutional Review Boards: A Time for Reform. Department of Health and Human Services, Office of Inspector General. 1998b Jun.

Brown, June Gibbs, Inspector General. Protecting Human Research Subjects: Status of Recommendations. Department of Health and Human Services, Office of Inspector General. April 2000.

Buckovich, Suzy A., Rippen, Helga E., and Rozen, Michael J. Driving Toward Guiding Principles: A Goal for Privacy, Confidentiality, and Security of Health Information. Journal of American Medical Informatics Association. 1999 Mar–1999 Apr 30; 6(2):123–133.

California Health Care Foundation. Americans Worry About the Privacy of Their Computerized Medical Reports. California Health Care Foundation: Communication— Press Releases. 1999 Jan 28.

Casarett, David; Karlawish Jason H.T., and Sugarman, Jeremy. Determining When Quality Improvement Intiatives Should Be Considered Research: Proposed Criteria and Potential Implications. JAMA. 2000 May 3; 283(17):2275–2280.

Chen, J.; Marciniak, T. A.; Radford, M. J.; Wang, Y., and Krumholz, H. M. Beta-blocker therapy for secondary prevention of myocardial infarction in elderly diabetic patients. Results from the National Cooperative Cardiovascular Project. Journal of the American College of Cardiology. 1999 Nov 1; 34(5):1388–1394.

Clancy, Carolyn M. and Eisenberg, John M. Outcomes Research; Measuring the End Results of Health Care. Science (Reprint Series). 1998 Oct 9; 282.

Cromwell, David M.; Bass, Eric B.; Steinberg, Earl P.; Yasui, Yutaka; Ravich, William J.; Hendrix, Thomas R.; McLeod, Susan F., and Moore, Richard D. Can Restrictions on Reimbursement for Anti-Ulcer Drugs Decrease Medicaid Pharmacy Costs Without Increasing Hospitalizations? Health Services Research; 33(6):1593–1610, 1999.

DHHS (Department of Health and Human Services), and Office of the Secretary. Standards for Privacy of Individually Identifiable Health Information; Proposed Rule. Federal Register. 1999 Nov 3; 64(212): 59918.

Edgar, Harold and Rothman, David J. The Institutional Review Board and Beyond: Future Challenges to the Ethics of Human Experimentation. The Milbank Quarterly. 1995; 73(4):489–506.

Eisenberg, John M. Health Services Research In A Market-Oriented Health Care System. Health Affairs Media & Managed Care. 1998 Jan–1998 Feb 28; 17(1).

Etzioni, Amitai. Medical Records: Enhancing Privacy, Preserving the Common Good. Hastings Center Report. 1999 Mar–1999 Apr 30:14–23.

General Accounting Office. Medical Records Privacy Access Needed for Health Research, but Oversight of Privacy Protections Is Limited. GAO—Report to Congressional Requesters. 1999 Feb., GAO/HEHS-99-55.

General Accounting Office. Scientific Research: Continued Vigilance Critical to protecting Human Subjects. GAO—Report to Ranking Minority Member. 1996 Mar., GAO/HEHS-96-72.

GHPP (Health Privacy Working Group). Best Principles for Health Privacy. Health Privacy Project; Institute for Health Care Research and Policy, Georgetown University.1999. Available online at http://www.healthprivacy.org/latest/Best_Principles_Report.pdf.

Goldman, Janlori, and Hudson, Zoe. A Health Privacy Primer for Consumers EXPOSED. Health Privacy Project. Institute for Health Care Research and Policy. Georgetown University. Washington, DC. 1999 Dec. Available online at http://www.healthprivacy.org/resources/exposed.pdf.

Goldman, Janlori. Protecting Privacy To Improve Health Care. Health Affairs. 1998 Nov–1998 Dec 31; 17(64):47–60.

Gostin, Lawrence O. and Hadley, Jack. Health Services Research: Public Benefits, Personal Privacy, and Proprietary Interests. Annals of Internal Medicine. 1998 Nov 15; 129(10):833–835.

Gostin, Lawrence O., Lazzarini, Zita; Neslund, Verla, and Osterholm, Michael T. The Public Health Information Infrastructure A National Review of the Law on Health Information Privacy. JAMA. 1996 Jun 26; 275(24):1921–1927.

Gross, David J.; Alecxih, Lisa; Gibson, Mary Jo; Corea, John; Caplan, Craig, and Brangan, Normandy. Out-of-Pocket Health Spending by Poor and Near-Poor Elderly Medicare Beneficiaries. Health Care Research Selected Papers From the Association For Health Services Research Annual Meeting, June 21–23, 1998. 1999 Apr; 34(1 Part II):241–254.

Halamka, John D.; Szolovits, Peter; Rind, David, and Safran, Charles. A WWW Implementation of National Recommendations for Protecting Electronic Health Information. Journal of the American Medical Informatics Association. 1997; 4(6):458–464.

Hanken, Mary Alice. Standards for Confidentiality, Privacy, Access, and Data Security. Topics in Health Information Management. 1996 May:44–48.

Iezzoni, Lisa. Ethical Consideration in Future Health Care Research: Protecting Privacy and Related Concerns. Presented at Connecting Ethics and Health Policy, Bethesda, Maryland, Oct 1, 1999.

Ivy, Andrew C. Nazi War Crimes of a Medical Nature. Reprinted With Permission of the Editors from Federation Bulletin. 1947; 33:133–146 in Reiser, Stanley J.; Dyke, Arthur J., and Curran, William J. Ethics in Medicine: Historical Perspectives and Contemporary Concerns. MIT Press. 1977.

IOM (Institute of Medicine). Committee on Regional Health Data Networks and Molla Donaldson, and Kathleen N. Lohr, editors. Health Data in the Information Age: Use, Disclosure, and Privacy. 1994. Washington, DC: National Academy Press.

IOM (Institute of Medicine). Committee on Health Services Research: Training and Work Force Issues and Marilyn J. Field, Robert E. Tranquada and Jill C. Feasley, editors. Health Services Research: Work. Washington, DC: National Academy Press. 1995.

ISPE (International Society for Pharmacoepidemiology). Data privacy, medical record confidentiality, and research in the interest of public health. [Web Page]. 1997 Sep 1. Available at: http://www.pharmacoepi.org/policy/privacy.htm.

JHITA (Joint Healthcare Information Technology Alliance). Advocacy Paper: Medical Records Confidentiality Legislation [Web Page]. Available at: http://www.jhita. org/medical.htm.

Katz, David A. Barriers Between Guidelines and Improved Patient Care: An Analysis of AHCPR's Unstable Angina Clinical Practice Guideline. Health Care Research Selected Papers From the Association For Health Services Research Annual Meeting, June 21–23, 1998. 1999 Apr; 34(1 Part II):377–389.

Kohane, Isaac S.; Dong, Hongmei, and Szolovits, Peter. Health Information Identification and De-Identification Toolkit. Proceedings of the American Medical Informatics Association, Symp. 1998; 356–360.

Lo, Bernard, and Alpers, Ann. Uses and Abuses of Prescription Drug Information in Pharmacy Benefits Management Programs. JAMA. 2000 Feb 9; 283(6):801–806.

Lo, Bernard. Values in Research: What are policy-relevant issues to study: How to do it ethically? Presented at Connecting Ethics and Health Policy, Bethesda, Maryland, Oct 1, 1999.

Lowrance, William W. Privacy and Health Research: A Report to the U.S. Secretary of Health and Human Services. 1997 May.

Malenka, D. J.; McGarth, P. D.; Wennberg, D. E.; Ryan, T. J Jr.; Kellett, M. A. Jr.; Shubrooks, S. J. Jr.; Bradley, W. A.; Hettelemen, B. D.; Robb, J. F.; Hearne, M. J.; Silver, T. M.; Watkins, M. W.; O'Meara, J. R.; VerLee, P. N., and O'Rourke, D. J. The relationship between operator volume and outcomes after percutaneous coronary interventions in high volume hospitals in 1994–1996: the northern New England experience. Northern New England Cardiovascular Disease Study Group. Journal of the American College of Cardiology. 1999 Nov 1; 34(5):1471–1480.

McCarthy, Douglas B.; Shatin, Deborah; Drinkard, Carol R.; Kleinman, John H., and Gardner, Jacqueline S. Medical Records and Privacy: Empirical Effects on Legislation. HSR: Health Services Research. 1999 Apr; 34 (part II)(1):417–425.

Melton, L. Joseph III. The Threat to Medical-Records Research. The New England Journal of Medicine. 1997 Nov 13; 337(20).

Norsigian, Judy and Billings, Paul. Privacy and Medical-Records Research. The New England Journal of Medicine. 1998 Apr 9; 338(15).

Norton, E. C.; Garfinkel, S. A.; McQuay, L. J.; Heck, D. A.; Wright, JG.; Dittus, R., and Lubitz, R.M. The effect of hospital volume on the in-hospital complication rate in knee replacement patients. Health Services Research. 1998 Dec; 33(5 Pt 1):1191–1210.

NRC (National Research Council). Committee on Maintaining Privacy and Security in Health Care Applications of the National Infrastructure, Computer Science and Telecommunications Board, Commission on Physical Sciences, Mathematics and Applications, and National Research Council. For the Record. Protecting Electronic Health Information. Washington, DC: National Academy Press. 1997.

NRC (National Research Council) Panel of Confidentiality and Data Access, George T. Duncan, Thomas B. Jabine, and Virginia A. de Wolf, editors. Private Lives and Public Policies Confidentiality and Accessibility of Government Statistics. 1993.

O'Brien, Dale G., and Yasnoff, William A. Privacy, Confidentiality, and Security in Information Systems of State Health Agencies. American Journal of Preventive Medicine. 1999; 16(4):351–358.

OPRR, National Institute of Health. Intitutional Review Board (IRB) Guidebook, 1993 [Web Page]. 1993. Available at: http://grants.nih.gov/grants/oprr/irb/irb_guidebook. htm.

PhRMA. PhRMA Policy Papers: Twin Goals: Privacy and Progress [Web Page]. Available at: http://www.phrma.org/issues/goals.html.

Pritts, J.; Goldman, J.; Hudson, Z.; Berenson, A.; and Hadley, E. The State of HealthPrivacy: An Uneven Terrain—A Comprehensive Survey of State Health Privacy Statutes. Health Privacy Project; Institute for Health Care Research and Policy, Georgetown University. 1999. Available online at http://www.healthprivacy.org/resources/statereports/contents.html

Shalala, Donna. Confidentiality of Individually Identifiable Health Information, Recommendations of the Secretary of Health and Human Services, pursuant to section 264 of the Health Insurance Portability and Accountability Act of 1996. 1997 Sep 11.

Sollano, J. A.; Gelijns, A. C.; Moskowitz, A. J.; Heitjan, D. F.; Cullinane, S.; Saha, T.; Chen, J. M.; Roohan, P. J.; Reemstsma, K.; and Shields, E. P. Volume-outcome relationships in cardiovascular operations: New York State, 1990–1995. Journal of Thoracic Cardiovascular Surgery. 1999 Mar; 117(3):419–428.

Sweeney, LaTanya. Weaving Technology and Policy Together to Maintain Confidentiality. Journal of Law, Medicine & Ethics. 1997; 25:98–110.

Ubel, PA; Zell, MM; Miller, DJ; Fischer, GS; Peters-Stefani, D; and Arnold, RM. Elevator talk: observational study of inappropriate comments in a public space. American Journal of Medicine. 1995; 99:190–194.

Wolf, Leslie E. and Lo, Bernard. Practicing Safer Research Using the Law to Protect the Confidentiality of Sensitive Research Data. IRB: A Review of Human Subjects Research, 1999; 21(5):4–7

Woodward, Beverly. Challenges to Human Subject Protections in US Medical Research. JAMA. 1999 Nov 24; 282(20):1947–1965.

Zito, Julie Magno; Safer, Daniel J.; dosReis, Susan; Gardner, James F.; Boles, Myde, and Lynch, Frances. Trends in the Prescribing of Psychotropic Medications to Preschoolers. JAMA. 2000 Feb 23; 283(8):1025–1030.

Acronyms and Abbreviations

AAMC	Association of American Medical Colleges
ACE	American College of Epidemiology
AHRQ	Agency for Healthcare Research and Quality
AHSR	Association for Health Services Research
ASPE	Assistant Secretary for Planning and Evaluation
ARENA	Applied Research Ethics National Association
ASPE	Assistant Secretary for Planning and Evaluation
CFR	Code of Federal Regulations
DHHS	Department of Health and Human Services
DSL	Digital Subscriber Line
FDA	Food and Drug Administration
GAO	General Accounting Office
GHPP	Georgetown Health Privacy Project
HIPAA	Health Insurance Portability and Accountability Act
HIV	Human Immunodeficiency Virus
HMO	Health Maintenance Organization
HSR	Health Services Research
IHC	Intermountain Health Care

IISC	IHC Information Security Committee
IOM	Institute of Medicine
IRB	Institutional Review Board
ISPE	International Society for Pharmacoepidemiology
IT	Information Technology
JHITA	Joint Healthcare Information Technology Alliance
MCWIRB	Medical College of Wisconsin IRB Discussion Forum
MPA	Multiple Project Assurance
NHIS	National Health Interview Survey
NIH	National Institutes of Health
NRC	National Research Council
OECD	Organization for Economic Cooperation and Development
OHRP	Office of Human Research Protections (formerly OPRR)
OIG	Office of Inspector General
OMB	Office of Management and Budget
OPRR	Office for Protection from Research Risks
PBM	Pharmacy Benefit Management
PhRMA	Pharmaceutical Research and Manufacturers of America
PKI	Public Key Infrastructure
PRIM&R	Public Responsibility in Medicine and Research
QA	Quality Assurance
QI	Quality Improvement
RTI	Research Triangle Institute
UCSF	University of California at San Francisco
USUHS	Uniform Services University of Health Sciences
UTHSCSA	University of Texas Health Sciences Center in San Antonio
WIRB	Western Institutional Review Board

APPENDIX A

Study Activities

As contracted with the sponsors, the Agency for Healthcare Research and Quality and the Office of the Assistant Secretary for Planning and Evaluation, the Institute of Medicine created a 12-person committee that was charged with identifying best practices of institutional review boards and private organizations in the protection of privacy and maintenance of confidentiality in health services research. The committee included members with expertise in medical ethics, health services research, epidemiological research, clinical research, IRB function, health and privacy law, statistics, computer science, and health database administration. The committee met by telephone conference call in January 2000 and held a workshop in March 2000 (agenda follows). The workshop, which was open to the public, included presentations from IRB administrators and chairs, research foundations, and health care services companies (see Appendix B). The workshop also featured presentations of the drafts of two commissioned papers (see Appendixes C and D). In addition to the workshop, the committee posted an invitation on a list serve and on the National Academies' website to IRBs to contribute information (invitation follows workshop agenda).

WORKSHOP ON INSTITUTIONAL REVIEW BOARDS

Institute of Medicine
Cecil and Ida Green Building,
Rooms GR-130 and GR-110
2001 Wisconsin Avenue, N.W.
March 13–14, 2000

Monday, March 13, 2000

8:30 a.m.   Call to Order, Welcome by Chair Bernard Lo, M.D.
                Charge to Committee, Introductions, Procedures, and
                    Greetings from Sponsors

9:15   OPRR overview
                Thomas Puglisi, Ph.D.

9:30   IRB Administrators
                Art Anderson, M.D., Fort Detrick, U.S. Army
                Angie Khan, University of Texas Health Science Center,
                    San Antonio

10:00   Discussion

10:30   Break

10:45   IRB Chairs/or Members
                James Kahn, M.D., University of California at San Francisco
                Robert Amdur, M.D., University of Florida
                Steve Garfinkel, Ph.D., Research Triangle Institute
                Tora Bikson, Ph.D., RAND Corporation

11:45   Discussion

12:30 p.m.   Lunch

1:30   Private/or Independent IRB
                Angela Bowen, M.D., Western Institutional Review Board

1:45   Discussion

2:00   Pharmaceutical Company
                Harry Guess, Ph.D., Merck

2:15   Discussion

2:30	Health Services Companies
	Fred Teitelbaum, Ph.D., and Jennifer Low, Esq.,
	Express Scripts
	Brent James, M.D., and Morris Linton, J.D., Intermountain
	Health Care
	Andrew Nelson, HealthPartners

| 3:15 | Discussion |

| 3:30 | BREAK |

| 3:45 | Comparing Privacy Standards Internationally |
| | Bartha Knoppers, J.D. |

| 4:15 | Discussion |

| 5:30 | Adjourn |

Tuesday, March 14 (GR 110)

| 8:30 a.m. | Call to Order, welcome by Chair, Brief Introductions of |
| | Committee |

| 9:00 | Technical Update |
| | Lawrence Dietz, Esq., Axent Technologies |

| 9:15 | Discussion |

| 9:30 | Special Considerations Regarding Data on Minors |
| | Ross Thompson, Ph.D. |

| 10:00 | Discussion |

| 10:15 | Break |

10:30	Special Considerations of Privacy in Heavily Studied
	Minority Populations
	William Freeman, M.D.

| 10:45 | Discussion |

| 11:00 | General Discussion |

| 12:00 noon | Adjourn Open Session |

INVITATION TO IRBS TO PROVIDE INFORMATION ON PRACTICES OF REVIEWING HEALTH SERVICES RESEARCH[*]

The Institute of Medicine (IOM) is conducting a project on the role of IRBs in the protection of data privacy in health services research. As part of that project, we are requesting general information from practitioners in the field with respect to the issues identified below. We expect that this information request will be of interest to those who currently chair, serve on, or administer an IRB, and whose committee at least occasionally receives protocols for research that depend on secondary data mining or linkage, in health services research or similar secondary analyses of health-related data.

By "health services research" we mean studies primarily using already-collected data to examine the impact of organization, financing, and management of health care services on access to, or the delivery, cost, outcomes, or quality of, services. Secondarily, we would include studies of already collected data that associate data sets to examine the outcomes of interventions, where similar privacy issues may arise.

Under the Statement of Task for this project, the IOM will gather information on current practices and principles, and if possible, recommend a set of best practices, for use by IRBs in safeguarding data privacy in health services research. The IOM has appointed a committee and has scheduled a workshop intended to supply information to the committee with respect to these issues.

Interested persons are invited to provide information regarding the practices of IRBs in protecting data privacy in health services research. This is not intended as a comprehensive survey, and we are not testing any specific hypothesis. Please feel free to elaborate on some or all of the issues identified below.

Unless you indicate otherwise on your response, your name and contact information will be made available only to IOM staff, and will not be presented to the study committee. The substance of your response (without your name and contact information) will be provided to the IOM study committee (with your response identified only by general category such as hospital, university, etc.) and will be included in a public access file created by the IOM and made available to the public upon request. By submitting a response, you give permission to the IOM to quote or use all or part of your submission (without specific identification of you) in our final report or other works of the institution, which may be posted on the world wide web or translated into other languages.

If you would like to provide information, please send it to the contact points below. Please also feel free, as always, to contact the Responsible IOM Staff Officer listed below if you wish to discuss any aspect of the project.

---

[*]Posted on MCWIRB list serve and National Academies Current Projects System website.

Discussion Issues

1. Policy or practices, if any, for identifying specific studies as health services research.

2. Procedures, if any, for determining which health services research studies are exempt from IRB review.

3. Procedures, if any, to determine whether and which information is identifiable when assessing risk of disclosure in an health services research protocol.

4. Procedures, if any, for weighing the importance of the research relative to the risk (of disclosure) to those whose data are used.

5. Procedures, if any, in place for merging different datasets, and in that context, for assuring that identifiable health information is protected

6. Procedures, if any, used for reviewing protocols to assure that identifiable health information is being protected while the study is actually underway.

7. Procedures, if any, to review protocols for the protection of data after a study is completed.

8. Procedures, if any, for auditing or oversight to make sure protections and procedures are used and enforced.

9. Provisions, procedures and/or principles that should be more widely adopted by IRBs in safeguarding data privacy in health services research.

Thank you.

Lee L. Zwanziger, Ph.D.
Senior Program Officer
Institute of Medicine

B

Institutional Review Boards and Health Services Research Data Privacy: A Workshop Summary

Executive Summary

The Institute of Medicine (IOM) and the Committee on the Role of Institutional Review Boards in Health Services Research Data Privacy Protection hosted a workshop on March 13–14, 2000, to gather and to exchange information on the protection of human subjects in health services research (HSR). HSR examines the impact of the organization, financing and management, of health care services, on the access to, delivery, cost, outcomes and quantity of those services. The benefits of such studies include increased understanding of the effects of changing parts of the health care system, such as whether a change in the reimbursement policy for a particular class of drug has any effect on the health or quality of life of the participants. The major risk in such research is not physical harm, but risk resulting from improper disclosure of personal information, that is, a breach of confidentiality. Confidentiality can be protected by limiting access to data and strengthening protections of data handling. However, HSR can be conducted only if researchers have access to data. Thus, data privacy and data access are objectives that have to be balanced.

POLICY CONTEXT

In recent years, public interest in and concern about the privacy of personally identifiable health information has increased. Currently, there is no comprehensive federal law that affords protection for the privacy of all health-related information. There are some federal laws, and state statutes varying by locale,

---

This Appendix was released as a separate workshop summary in June 2000.

that protect certain types of personally identifiable health information under certain circumstances (Gostin et al., 1996; O'Brian and Yasnoff, 1999; Goldman and Hudson, 1999).

In 1996, Congress enacted the Health Insurance Portability and Accountability Act (HIPAA), which directed the Secretary of Health and Human Services to publish regulations by February 2000, unless the Congress had taken legislative action at least six months earlier. The Secretary published a Notice of Proposed Rulemaking in November 1999 (Department of Health and Human Services, 1999), with the comment period closing on February 17, 2000. As this workshop was being held and summarized, the Department was analyzing and responding to the many (approximately 52,000) comments that the proposed rule elicited.

Historically, the focus of institutional review boards (IRBs) has been on protecting human subjects from harm associated with invasive clinical procedures or administration of new drugs. In HSR there are few physical risks. Much HSR involves the analysis of previously collected, personally identifiable, health information recorded in the course of clinical care, billing, or payment for services. Thus, in HSR the primary risks are due to breaches of confidentiality, with ensuing loss of privacy and possible stigma and discrimination. Little is known about IRB practices in the area of HSR projects. Furthermore, much HSR using large databases falls outside the scope of federal regulations that require oversight by IRBs because it is undertaken with private funding by organizations that do not hold federal multiproject assurances that require all research at the institution to fall under IRB review.

SCOPE OF PROJECT

In order to facilitate the national discussion of the topic of IRB oversight of HSR, the sponsors commissioned the IOM to call together a panel of national experts on various aspects of the problem. The purpose of this project was to provide information and advice on the current and best practices of IRBs in protecting privacy in health services research. The project was sponsored by the Agency for Healthcare Research and Quality and the Office of the Assistant Secretary for Planning and Evaluation, both in the Department of Health and Human Services. The charge to the committee was as follows:

1. To gather information on the current practices and principles followed by institutional review boards to safeguard the confidentiality of personally identifiable health information used for health services research purposes, in particular, to identify those IRB practices that are superior in protecting the privacy, confidentiality, and security of personally identifiable health information.

2. To gather information on the current practices and principles employed in privately funded health services research studies (that are generally not subject to IRB approval) to safeguard the confidentiality of personally identifiable

health information, and to consider whether and how IRB best practices in this regard might be applied to such privately sponsored studies.

3. If appropriate, to recommend a set of best practices for safeguarding the confidentiality of personally identifiable health information that might be voluntarily applied to health services research projects by IRBs and private sponsors.

This summary describes the presentations and discussions that took place at the IOM Workshop on the role of Institutional Review Boards and Health Services Research Data Privacy. This summary reflects what transpired at the workshop and does not include committee deliberations, findings, or conclusions. The committee's deliberative report is being published separately (IOM, 2000).

WORKSHOP

The workshop itself was one of the major information-gathering activities of the committee. The committee invited speakers including IRB administrators and chairs from universities, research foundations, the U.S. Army and private businesses, as well as representatives from health care services and pharmaceutical companies. The committee also welcomed all interested parties to attend and to participate in discussion periods following the presentations. The invited speakers and members of the audience were asked to provide information on what their organizations actually do to protect confidentiality in health services research, whether or not the research they do falls under the purview of the common rule. The committee also asked the participants to share any observations they had made regarding which practices are best and which might be applicable to other institutions.

The Office for Protection from Research Risks (OPRR) is the agency that administers the federal regulations on human and animal subjects. The director of OPRR's Division on Human Subject Protections presented an overview of federal regulations on human subjects, particularly regulations pertaining to the determination of whether a records review study involves human subjects, when data are considered identifiable, whether a study might be exempted from IRB review, and whether informed consent from subjects might be waived.

The committee heard presentations by several speakers who administer or chair IRBs in universities, private foundations, corporations, or military settings. Highlights mentioned included how IRBs have wrestled with determining whether data would be identifiable and how to ensure that potential risks to all affected parties are considered. For instance, the set of subjects may include not only the patients who received a service, but also the health care providers who delivered the service. In most HSR studies, the subjects themselves are not likely to receive any direct benefit, so the tolerance of some IRBs for risk to the subjects is correspondingly low, although IRBs consider risk to subjects in balance with the benefits to society of the research in the case of HSR as with any protocol. Other highlights follow.

An IRB chair from the UCSF medical school reported on an internal study leading to a recommendation that research grants should include 1.0 to 1.5 percent of the budget as an above-the-line item directed to the support of the institution's human subjects protection program.

A former IRB chair, recently relocated to University of Florida, identified the differentiation of health services research and health services operations as critical, but also noted that the evaluation of risks to privacy is not new for IRBs and that current federal regulations allow appropriate flexibility.

An IRB chair from RAND described its on-line system for initiating research projects, designed to help investigators determine whether the project might be addressed as research and, if so, to explore the possibilities of exemption from full IRB review, eligibility for expedited review, or requirement for full review. This IRB has access to a three-person privacy team, including an information resource specialist, a data librarian, and a networks specialist, to help design and implement data safeguarding plans commensurate with the level of risk for various protocols.

An IRB chair from the Research Triangle Institute observed that it is very important that health services researchers have the freedom to work with their IRBs to modify standard consent and confidentiality language as appropriate for the particular study in question. He concluded that although many issues are often not well understood by IRB members or by researchers because they represent new or rare situations, the IRB system is workable and working, and has never in his experience been an onerous burden to researchers.

An officer from Intermountain Health Care described the comprehensive technical protections and enforceable policies the organization has implemented in the protection of personally identifiable health information, whether in the context of research or in day to day operations of providing health services. He noted that all known violations of privacy have occurred in operations, but none have been found in the research branch.

A representative of AXENT, an information security firm, spoke on recent market trends in security such as the widespread adoption of Web access security products and virtual private networks, the slower adoption of products for authenticating users (i.e., public key infrastructure products), public key infrastructure products, and the general tendency of organizations to contract for information technologists rather than develop in-house expertise.

The chair of the IRB of the Indian Health Service spoke about ethical issues regarding research with minority groups, including both the privacy of individuals within small and isolated groups and the privacy of the group itself. In either case, he observed, consultation with individuals familiar with the particulars of the group is important to avoid unintentional privacy violations and to build trust between the researchers and the participants.

The committee had commissioned two background papers, in accord with the contract between the IOM and the sponsors, which were presented in draft at the workshop. One paper analyzed issues regarding HSR with children. The author identified three issues of particular concern in considering health services research involving minors, including the heterogeneity of the population in question, complications arising from proxy consent, and the changing interests and risks affecting the subjects as they grow older. The second commissioned paper analyzed international standards regarding the use of personally identifiable health information for HSR. The author studied international conventions and guidelines and the domestic law of several nation states. This analysis pointed out different approaches to requiring oversight of the use of personally identifiable health information in HSR by IRB-like bodies and the uses of such information without individual consent. Both papers are appended to the committee's report, as is this workshop summary.

1

Introduction

The Institute of Medicine and the Committee on the Role of Institutional Review Boards in Health Services Research Data Privacy Protection hosted a workshop on March 13–14, 2000, to gather and to exchange information on human subjects protection in health services research.

Health services research uses quantitative or qualitative methodology to examine the impact of the organization, financing, and management of health care services on the access to and the delivery, cost, outcomes, and quality of services. Another IOM committee (IOM, 1995) recently developed the following definition:

> Health services research is a multidisciplinary field of inquiry, both basic and applied, that examines the use, costs, quality, accessibility, delivery, organization, financing, and outcomes of health care services to increase knowledge and understanding of the structure, processes, and effects of health services for individuals and populations.

As these definitions show, HSR includes a broad range of questions and of research methodologies. This IOM project concentrates on HSR conducted through analyses of previously existing databases of health information. Further, among such studies, this project considers just the role of institutional review boards in ensuring that the study design will maintain confidentiality in the use of the subjects' data.

The benefits of HSR studies include increased understanding of the results of policy changes and other systemic effects in health care. The major risk in this branch of research, where the actual object of study is not the human body, but data about human beings, is likewise not to life and limb, but rather the risk resulting from improper disclosure of personal information. Any potential for harm would come about through possible breaches of confidentiality. The methodology, and in many respects the type of questions, of HSR are often very similar to the questions and methods directed toward assessing and improving the quality of operations within an organization. As a result, a boundary between research and operations is often difficult to locate.

It is important to distinguish privacy and confidentiality. The following explanation is provided by the Office of Protection from Research Risks in guidance to institutional review boards.

> Privacy can be defined in terms of having control over the extent, timing, and circumstances of sharing oneself (physically, behaviorally, or intellectually) with others. Confidentiality pertains to the treatment of information that an individual has disclosed in a relationship of trust and with the expectation that it will not be divulged to others in ways that are inconsistent with the understanding of the original disclosure without permission. (OPRR Guidebook, Chapter Three, Section D, 1993)

The protection of privacy is an important matter, and many individuals regard the protection of their privacy (and likewise the confidential treatment of private information they choose to disclose) as an important ethical value. The responsible conduct of high-quality research is also an important value, and many individuals appreciate the benefits of effective health care, efficacy that is based on information that can be obtained only from population data. Privacy and confidentiality can be protected by limiting access to data. Good research can be conducted only if investigators have access to data. Risks to individuals (from possible breaches of confidentiality) and benefits both to individuals and society (from the results of good research) are thus two concerns that we must balance.

In research, one way to ensure that subjects are protected, and in particular for this report's concerns, that the confidentiality of personally identifiable health information is maintained, is to have the proposed study reviewed by an institutional review board (IRB). IRBs are usually located within the organization doing the research, so that they can be aware of the nuances of the local situation. IRBs must ensure that they follow federal regulations pertaining to the protection of human subjects but they also use their local knowledge in practice along with the general principles in those regulations. This is why it was important in this project to consider the practices that IRBs actually follow as well as the regulations they apply through those practices.

It is also important to understand that IRB review is required only for research activities. So if data were to be collected for some proposed research (i.e., federally funded or otherwise subject to federal regulation), the protocol would be reviewed by an IRB for the protection of confidentiality. But health care provider or product companies often undertake reviews of their internal operations to assess and improve the quality of care and/or products they provide. These quality assessment and quality improvement exercises are not defined as research but may involve similar types of data collection as HSR, as well as raising similar questions about the use of private information and the maintenance of confidentiality. So if similar data were to be collected or used by a health care provider or health product company in the course of day-to-day clinical care or business operations, such collection and use would not be subject to regulations requiring IRB review.

BACKGROUND AND POLICY CONTEXT

In recent years, public interest in and concern about privacy and personally identifiable health information has increased and continues (e.g., Appelbaum, 2000). Some individuals have been disturbed, for instance, at corporate use of health information to create targeted mailings that seem to straddle the line between anticipating health questions and marketing products. For example, a database marketing firm received patient prescription records from two large pharmacies in the Washington, D.C. metro area (Lo and Alpers, 2000). The firm then created mailings for the pharmacies on the pharmacies' letterhead targeted to consumers of certain prescription drug products, informing them of new products with similar indications. The project, which was quickly canceled by the pharmacies in response to customer complaints, had been sponsored by the manufacturers of the new products, although the manufacturers never had access to any patient records themselves. In other cases, these worries have been heightened by still more dramatic reports of privacy violations, such as the release of HIV test results of hundreds of individuals to several Florida newspapers (in Etzioni, 1999). Such incidents are not HSR, but still increase general concern about the reliability of privacy protections.

In 1996, Congress enacted the Health Insurance Portability and Accountability Act directing the Secretary of Health and Human Services to prepare detailed recommendations on standards for privacy and personally identifiable health information. The Secretary's recommendations were delivered to Congress in September 1997 (Shalala, 1997), and several privacy bills have been introduced in Congress since that time. Both the Secretary's recommendations and most of the privacy bills introduced in the 105th Congress would permit personally identifiable health information to be used in research without the person's explicit permission if the research project were approved by an IRB.

The HIPAA further directed the Secretary of Health and Human Services to publish regulations on privacy standards by February 2000, unless the Congress had taken legislative action at least six months earlier. The Secretary published a Notice of Proposed Rulemaking in November 1999, with the comment period closing on February 17, 2000 (Department of Health and Human Services, 1999). The proposed regulations would create new requirements for privacy protection for all health care providers and health plans, and would establish research standards and oversight for all research. In addition, the proposed rule would permit the use and disclosure of personally identifiable health information for research without authorization by the subject, as long as the research protocol had been approved by an IRB or, if it does not fall under regulations requiring IRB review, then by an equivalent body. As this workshop was being held and summarized, the department was analyzing and responding to the many (approximately 52,000) comments that the proposed rule elicited.

Another important context for this report is recent media attention to research on human subjects. For example, news stories on topics such as gene therapy and clinical trials in developing countries have highlighted concerns about human subjects protections. Policies on many levels, from institutional to international, address of the proper and ethical conduct of research with human subjects. In the United States, the use of human beings as research subjects is governed by federal regulations when the research is federally funded. The body of federal regulations about human subjects protection (45 CFR 46 Subpart A) is called the Common Rule, since it has been adopted "in common" by many federal departments and agencies that are involved in research with human subjects as the basis for their regulations. The Food and Drug Administration (FDA) has adopted similar regulations (21 CFR 50 and 56) and will not consider clinical trial results submitted in support of a marketing application unless the trial was approved by an IRB. In addition, many organizations that do human subjects research have entered into agreements to conduct all their research according to the Common Rule, regardless of funding. Such agreements are called multiple product assurances (MPAs, see also footnote 6 below).

The provisions of this shared body of regulation, including the Common Rule and MPAs as well as FDA regulations, grew from a variety of sources including the Belmont Report (Belmont, 1979). The Belmont Report presented the ethical basis of human subjects research as three principles: respect for persons, beneficence, and justice. The main mechanism in the human subjects protection system for protecting research subjects and for assessing the balance between the risks and benefits of research is the institutional review board. An IRB is a standing committee composed of scientists and/or physicians not directly involved with the proposal being reviewed and including at least one person who is not primarily involved in scientific pursuits and at least one person who is not otherwise connected with the institution. IRBs review proposals for research with human participants to make sure that any risk of harm to the subjects of the research is reasonable in relation to the possible benefits and that they will be respected as persons, not just used as research subjects. In many studies the subjects participate only after giving informed consent. So the IRB must make sure that subjects will be fully informed and then have an opportunity to consent, decline to participate in the research, or withdraw at anytime, unless the research is of such low risk that informed consent is not needed. In federal regulations, the IRB of a particular organization is charged with reviewing and approving all research at the institution covered by the regulations. The criteria set out in the regulations for IRBs to use in assessing research proposals are listed in Box 1-1.

BOX 1-1 Criteria for IRB Approval of Research

Sec. 46.111 Criteria for IRB approval of research.

(a) In order to approve research covered by this policy the IRB shall determine that all of the following requirements are satisfied:

(1) Risks to subjects are minimized: (i) By using procedures which are consistent with sound research design and which do not unnecessarily expose subjects to risk, and (ii) whenever appropriate, by using procedures already being performed on the subjects for diagnostic or treatment purposes.

(2) Risks to subjects are reasonable in relation to anticipated benefits, if any, to subjects, and the importance of the knowledge that may reasonably be expected to result. In evaluating risks and benefits, the IRB should consider only those risks and benefits that may result from the research (as distinguished from risks and benefits of therapies subjects would receive even if not participating in the research). The IRB should not consider possible long-range effects of applying knowledge gained in the research (for example, the possible effects of the research on public policy) as among those research risks that fall within the purview of its responsibility.

(3) Selection of subjects is equitable. In making this assessment the IRB should take into account the purposes of the research and the setting in which the research will be conducted and should be particularly cognizant of the special problems of research involving vulnerable populations, such as children, prisoners, pregnant women, mentally disabled persons, or economically or educationally disadvantaged persons.

(4) Informed consent will be sought from each prospective subject or the subject's legally authorized representative, in accordance with, and to the extent required by Sec. 46.116.

(5) Informed consent will be appropriately documented, in accordance with, and to the extent required by Sec. 46.117.

(6) When appropriate, the research plan makes adequate provision for monitoring the data collected to ensure the safety of subjects.

(7) When appropriate, there are adequate provisions to protect the privacy of subjects and to maintain the confidentiality of data.

(b) When some or all of the subjects are likely to be vulnerable to coercion or undue influence, such as children, prisoners, pregnant women, mentally disabled persons, or economically or educationally disadvantaged persons, additional safeguards have been included in the study to protect the rights and welfare of these subjects.

SOURCE: 45 CFR 46, Subpart A 46.111.

Research using databases containing health information on individuals, of which health services research is one example, also falls under the Common Rule, although the Belmont Report and regulations primarily address clinical research and individual direct interventions. HSR involving the analysis of previously collected data is somewhat different from clinical research in that subjects participate indirectly because researchers are sorting data on large sets of individuals but not intervening with the specific individuals themselves. As a result, the application of the principles may also have to be somewhat different in HSR.

PROJECT OBJECTIVES

The sponsors commissioned the IOM to call together a panel of national experts on various aspects of the problem. The purpose of this project was to provide information and advice on the current and best practices of IRBs in protecting confidentiality in health services research. The project was sponsored by the Agency for Healthcare Research and Quality and the Office of the Assistant Secretary for Planning and Evaluation, both in the Department of Health and Human Services.

The charge to the committee was as follows:

1. To gather information on the current practices and principles followed by institutional review boards to safeguard the confidentiality of personally identifiable health information used for health services research purposes, in particular, to identify those IRB practices that are superior in protecting the privacy, confidentiality, and security of personally identifiable health information.

2. To gather information on the current practices and principles employed in privately funded health services research studies (that are generally not subject to IRB approval) to safeguard the confidentiality of personally identifiable health information, and to consider whether and how IRB best practices in this regard might be applied to such privately sponsored studies.

3. If appropriate, to recommend a set of best practices for safeguarding the confidentiality of personally identifiable health information that might be voluntarily applied to health services research projects by IRBs and private sponsors.

The charge did not encompass many other possible questions about privacy of medical records or electronic records in general. The committee recognized the strong connections between these related matters and the question of protecting data confidentiality in health services research. However, in keeping with the committee's charge, these issues were not discussed at the workshop. The committee also did not discuss issues of privacy and confidentiality as they pertain to other types of research, for example, clinical research that deals with sensitive topics such as HIV infection, mental illness, or substance abuse.

The committee focused its attention on HSR involving the secondary analysis of existing data because this type of research raises the most dilemmas about how IRBs can protect the confidentiality of the patients' data. To be sure, HSR that involves, for example, questionnaires to patients about satisfaction or clinical outcomes also raises concerns about privacy and confidentiality. However, patients must be contacted and must cooperate for data to be gathered. Because of these interactions, the research may be less likely to be exempt from IRB review, and potential subjects have the ability to decline to participate. The committee therefore urges the reader to bear in mind that such related matters were not in the charge, were not addressed by the committee, and in particular, were not discussed at the workshop.

SCOPE OF WORKSHOP REPORT

This summary describes the presentations and discussions that took place at the March 13–14, 2000 IOM Workshop on Institutional Review Boards and Health Services Research Data Privacy Protection. This summary reflects what transpired at the workshop and does not include committee deliberations, findings or conclusions. The committee's deliberative report is being published separately (IOM, 2000).

The workshop itself was one of the major information-gathering activities of the committee. The committee invited speakers including IRB administrators and chairs from universities, research foundations, the U.S. Army, and private businesses, as well as representatives from health care services and pharmaceutical companies (see appended workshop agenda). The committee also welcomed all interested parties to attend and to participate in discussion periods following the presentations. The invited speakers and the audience were asked to provide information on what their organizations, whether IRBs or organizations doing research not under the purview of the Common Rule, currently and actually do to protect privacy in health services research. The committee also asked the participants to share any observations they had made regarding which practices are best and might be applicable to other institutions.

Some of the issues discussed at the workshop and in this document have been the subject of recent IOM and National Research Council (NRC) reports. These reports include *For the Record* (NRC, 1997), *Health Data in the Information Age* (IOM, 1994), and *Private Lives and Public Policies* (NRC, 1993).

DEFINITIONS

This summary uses several terms repeatedly, for which the committee has offered definitions below.[*] In most cases, these definitions are incomplete in a global sense, reflecting their use in the context of the present study; "privacy," for instance, has other shades of meaning to be sure, but the definition below emphasizes the use of the word in regard to information.

Informational Privacy—The right of individuals to control access to, and the use of, information about themselves.

---

[*]Bradburn, N., 2000; Buckovich et al., 1999; NRC, 1997; Lowrance, 1997; IOM, 1995; OPRR, 1993.

Confidential—a manner of treating private information, which has been disclosed by the individual subject of the information to a particular person or persons, such that further disclosure of the information will not be allowed to occur without authorization.

Health Services Research—a multidisciplinary field of inquiry, both basic and applied, that examines the use, costs, quality, accessibility, delivery, organization, financing, and outcomes of health care services to increase knowledge and understanding of the structure, processes, and effects of health services for individuals and populations.

Personally Identifiable Health Information—information such that an individual person can be identified as the subject.

Institutional Review Board—administrative body established to protect the rights and welfare of human research subjects in research activities of the institution to which the board is affiliated, by reviewing proposed research protocols and approving or requesting changes prior to their inception.

2

Workshop Summary

The Committee on the Role of Institutional Review Boards in Health Services Research Data Privacy Protection hosted a public workshop on March 13–14, 2000 (agenda appended). The committee invited speakers with a variety of institutional perspectives and also welcomed contributions from the audience. As a starting point for the workshop, the committee reviewed its charge (as given in the previous section). The committee was charged with collecting information on the current practices of institutional review boards for protecting data privacy in health services research, gathering information on the practices of organizations that are not required to consult IRBs but still carry out HSR activities where data privacy and confidentiality are of concern, and to the extent possible, identifying and recommending the best practices for wider adoption. This section presents a summary of the workshop proceedings. The summary does not include deliberations, findings, or recommendations by the committee (see IOM, 2000)

INTRODUCTORY PRESENTATIONS

The first series of presentations was given by representatives of several agencies within the federal Department of Health and Human Services (DHHS). The sponsors of the project, the Agency for Healthcare Research and Quality (AHRQ) and the Office of the Assistant Secretary for Planning and Evaluation (ASPE), outlined their perspective on the objectives of the workshop and the committee's task, and the Office for Protection from Research Risks (OPRR) provided an overview of the current regulations on the protection of human subjects in research.

Comments from Sponsoring Agencies

Dr. Michael Fitzmaurice of the AHRQ, one of the agencies sponsoring the project, spoke first. Dr. Fitzmaurice observed that the tension between the availability of data for research and the protection of data for maintaining confidentiality and privacy will not disappear but has to be managed through judicious balancing of these countervailing interests. Essentially, these interests should reinforce each other. In order to facilitate the national discussion of this balancing with regard to the use of individually identifiable health data by health services researchers with principles and best practices for maintaining confidentiality, the sponsors commissioned the Institute of Medicine (IOM) to convene a panel of national experts on various aspects of the problem. The panel's report will provide guidance to assist IRBs that review HSR, organizations that are not required to use IRBs but may still be concerned with balancing privacy and data access in such research, and health services researchers themselves.

Dr. Fitzmaurice continued that the DHHS is directed under the Health Insurance Portability and Accountability Act to promulgate federal regulations governing the privacy of personal health information. The proposed regulations allow the release of individually identifiable health data and information for use in research, under appropriate conditions. Current and proposed regulations would set conditions for safeguards that researchers must observe. Oversight mechanisms described in the proposed federal regulations on health privacy (Department of Health and Human Services, 1999) depend on the current IRB system but also would require complementary oversight bodies, called "privacy boards"(see Box 2-1); that would oversee the protection of personal health information in research not covered (by regulation or voluntarily) by the current IRB system—non-federally funded research for the most part.

Mr. John Fanning of the ASPE (also a sponsor of the project) provided further context for the workshop. Mr. Fanning pointed out that many sets of principles pertaining to privacy protection have already been published, but these principles may fail to provide practical guidance to investigators and IRBs concerned with HSR.[1] In addition, he noted, little information is available regarding actual practices and procedures whereby the principles are implemented by IRBs. Such information is needed in order for IRBs to improve their oversight of HSR. In particular, Mr. Fanning explained, the agencies sponsoring the project

---

[1]Because different groups are developing principles to address different problems, or at least to address problems in different contexts, the sets of principles do not directly overlap in many instances—in particular, not mentioning a principle is not evidence that an organization would oppose it. These different perspectives make for difficult comparison (though see Buckovich, 1999). See, for example, GHPP, 1999; ISPE, 1997; Lowrance, 1997; AAMC, 1997; JHITA (web page), PhRMA (web page).

BOX 2-1 Privacy Board Review of Research in the Proposed Rule

Privacy boards, in the proposed rule, would review the protocols for research proposing to use or disclose protected health information without individual authorization that does not fall under the Common Rule to determine that the research meets specified criteria. The board could be an IRB constituted under the Common Rule, or an equivalent privacy board that meets the requirements in this proposed rule (note that not all commentors agree that the board described would in fact be equivalent to an IRB). The criteria proposed were the following:

- the use or disclosure of protected health information involves no more than minimal risk to the subjects;
- the waiver or alteration will not adversely affect the rights and welfare of the subjects;
- the research could not practicably be carried out without the waiver or alteration;
- whenever appropriate, the subjects will be provided with additional pertinent information after participation;
- the research would be impracticable to conduct without the protected health information;
- the research project is of sufficient importance to outweigh the intrusion into the privacy of the individual whose information would be disclosed;
- there is an adequate plan to protect the identifiers from improper use and disclosure; and
- there is an adequate plan to destroy the identifiers at the earliest opportunity consistent with conduct of the research, unless there is a health or research justification for retaining the identifiers.

SOURCE: DHHS, 1999.

---

believe that identification of best practices of IRBs in reviewing HSR could provide helpful guidance to other IRBs, as well as to organizations that are not required to have IRBs review health services research but wish to ensure that confidentiality and privacy are adequately protected in HSR.

The location of the boundaries of HSR, in the focus of the present project, has been an additional and difficult question. The regulations now in place define "research" as an activity intended to result in generalizable knowledge. However, it is often difficult to draw a line between HSR and other activities that use personal health information in databases, such as internal efforts at quality assurance, business planning, or marketing.

In the discussion immediately following the presentations, committee members highlighted their concerns about focusing on the protection of privacy in the context of research while ignoring very similar activities using databases that contain personal health information when undertaken for business or administrative purposes. The sponsors' representatives replied that the Common Rule applies only to the oversight of research, not to these other activities. Thus, although the appropriate use of personal health information for purposes other than research is an important question that the nation has to address, the current project is intended to address only the more limited but still important topic of HSR.

Overview of Current Human Subjects Regulations

The OPRR administers the federal regulations on human and animal subjects. Dr. Thomas Puglisi, director of OPRR's Division of Human Subject Protections, presented an overview of the human subjects regulations to the committee. IRBs have to address several questions, all of which may require some interpretation specific to HSR. First, does an activity constitute research? Second, is the project exempt from IRB review? Third, may individual informed consent be waived?

Dr. Puglisi explained that the regulations apply to projects involving human subjects, defined as protocols in which there is to be an intervention or interaction with a living person that would not be occurring, or would be occurring in some other fashion, but for the research or if identifiable private data or information will be obtained for the protocol in a form associable with the individual (Figure 2-1). Private information, in this context, is defined as "information about behavior that occurs in a context in which an individual can reasonably expect that no observation or recording is taking place, and information which has been provided for specific purposes by an individual and which the individual can reasonably expect will not be made public (e.g. a medical record)" (45 CFR 46 102(f)). The definition stipulates that the information must be individually identifiable, that is, that the identity of the individual can be readily ascertained or associated with the information.

Dr. Puglisi noted that several aspects of these regulations already merit attention with regard to HSR. With HSR, the second condition marking an activity as research is generally the most pertinent ("identifiable private data or information will be obtained for the protocol in a form associable with the individual"), since HSR often works with data that have already been collected and hence requires no further interaction with subjects. The question of identifiability can be difficult, since coded data are not necessarily nonidentifiable because subjects often still can be identified by inference.

The term research is also defined in the regulations: the activity must be systematic and designed to contribute to generalizable knowledge. The important term "generalizable" is not, he pointed out, itself defined in the regulation. This term usually must mean at least that the product of the activity is intended to be applicable beyond the immediate situation and present conditions. For example, a project that is intended for publication in a medical journal or presentation at a conference would be deemed research, whereas an organization's internal review of records for the purpose of improving its operations would likely not be consid-

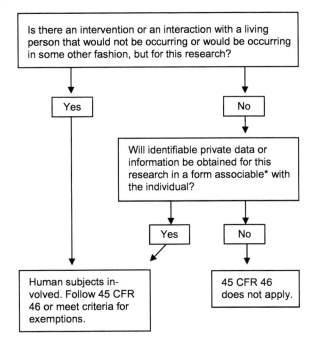

*That is, the identity of the
subject is associated with or
may readily be ascertained
form the information.

FIGURE 2-1 Is the definition of "human subject" at 45 CFR
46.102(f) met in the research activity?

ered research. Different organizations, however, make different distinctions between research and quality assurance activities.

Activities may be exempt from IRB review, either because they are not research or because they may not meet the definition of human subjects research
as described above. These conditions are a basis of a specific exemption (45
CFR 46.101(b)(4)):

> (4) Research involving the collection or study of existing data, documents, rec-
> ords, pathological specimens, or diagnostic specimens, if these sources are
> publicly available or if the information is recorded by the investigator in such a
> manner that subjects cannot be identified, directly or through identifiers linked
> to the subjects.

For a project that is research involving human subjects and is not eligible
for exemption as above, the IRB must ensure that the subjects have given free
and informed consent to participate, unless the informed consent requirement

can be waived. The requirement for informed consent may be waived by the IRB under some conditions including that the research involves no more than minimal risk and the research could not otherwise be practicably carried out (where "not practicable" is not specifically defined but means a general zone between merely inconvenient and truly impossible). The key point in considering when a waiver of informed consent would be appropriate is "minimal risk." In HSR, Dr. Puglisi explained, the IRB would have to consider the protections for confidentiality that were built into the protocol, keeping in mind that the protocol may require access to records on very large numbers of individuals, and weigh the probabilities of harm or wrong to these individuals. With adequate protections, the IRB often determines that the risk would be minimal and individual informed consent therefore unnecessary.

In discussion following the presentation, several committee members raised the question of review of a protocol's expected benefit to society and its scientific merit, with regard to which matter different IRBs take different views. The question of the role of OPRR in education also surfaced, in particular its possible involvement in collecting and disseminating information about the best practices of IRBs. Dr. Puglisi said that a great deal of information and guidance is posted on OPRR's website and that OPRR is actively expanding its educational activities.

IRB FUNCTION

Many different types of institutions conduct research with human subjects and therefore have IRBs associated with them, including universities, state and federal agencies, hospitals, and research foundations. The committee invited speakers from a variety of these institutions to present information on the practices and experience with protecting the confidentiality of data in health services research in their respective organizations.

In preparation for the workshop, the speakers were given a list of points to discuss points about IRBs and HSR, which are listed in Box 2-2.[2] Many presenters used these discussion points as a basis for their remarks. The summary of the presentations and discussion below follows these points as much as possible. Some discussion points, however, did not apply to some speakers, and several speakers remarked that they did not wish to repeat what had already been said about IRB function, so they did not specifically speak to all the discussion issues in their presentations.

---

[2]This list of suggested discussion issues was also posted on an IRB-targeted list serve and on the projects' section of the National Academies' Current Project System website, with an invitation to provide any relevant information or experience. The full invitation is included in Appendix A of IOM (2000).

BOX 2-2 Points to Discuss Regarding IRB Review of HSR

Policy or practices, if any, for identifying specific studies as health services research.

Procedures, if any, for determining which health services research studies are exempt from IRB review.

Procedures, if any, to determine whether and which information is identifiable when assessing risk of disclosure in a health services research protocol.

Procedures, if any, for weighing the importance of the research relative to the risk (of disclosure) to those whose data are used.

Procedures, if any, in place for merging different datasets and, in this context, for ensuring that identifiable health information is protected.

Procedures, if any, used for reviewing protocols to ensure that identifiable health information is being protected while the study is actually under way.

Procedures, if any, to review protocols for the protection of data after a study is completed.

Procedures, if any, for auditing or oversight to make sure protections and procedures are used and enforced.

Provisions, procedures, and/or principles that should be more widely adopted by IRBs in safeguarding data privacy in health services research.

SOURCE: IOM 2000, Appendix A.

IRB Administrators

The first speakers were IRB administrators. IRB administrators coordinate IRB activities and provide staff support for IRB meetings and actions. IRB administrators typically work very closely with their IRBs in substantive as well as procedural capacities, often serving as voting members and in some cases even chairing the board.

The first presenter was S. Angela Khan, Institutional Coordinator of Research Review of the IRB at the University of Texas Health Sciences Center in San Antonio (UTHSCSA). The second presenter was Colonel Arthur Anderson, M.D., administrator and also chair of the IRB for the U.S. Army Medical Research Institute of Infectious Diseases at Fort Detrick. Col. Anderson highlighted some of the special features of human subjects research in the military. The summary of their remarks follows, with some modifications, the issues listed in Box 2-2.

Identifying Specific Studies as HSR

Ms. Khan explained that the UTHSCSA IRB does not specifically classify protocols as to whether they are HSR, but in any case does not review such projects any differently than other protocols. This IRB has reviewed protocols addressing various HSR questions including the effects of training and of guidelines, the delivery and perception of services, and the costs of different services.

Col. Anderson explained that his institute is a research institute that is not primarily involved with providing health care to persons with illnesses. The institute does very little that would be classed as HSR but is heavily involved in vaccine research studies, which give rise to many concerns about privacy protections for the soldiers who volunteer.

Determining Which HSR Studies Qualify as Exempt

Ms. Khan reported that in assessing whether certain studies (generally only those directed toward internal quality assurance [QA]) should be exempt from review, the IRB would consider

- whether the findings of the study will be disseminated beyond the department proposing to carry out the study,
- whether the protocol includes any change in clinical care or clinical processes,
- whether the data to be collected would be available to the investigator only through the study (i.e., the investigator would not have access to such data in normal practice), and finally
- whether there is any risk to patients or staff.

If the answer to all these questions is no, then the protocol could be considered exempt as a QA activity. Other research may fall into an exempt category under the regulations but probably also would be reviewed at least by a subcommittee of the IRB, and informed consent might still be required. Ms. Khan also noted that generally the first consideration about publication is sufficient to classify a project as research since most investigators do in fact wish to publish their findings, even from projects that were planned as internal investigations, if they should prove interesting.

Ms. Khan explained that other research that falls into one of the categories defined in the regulations as exempt undergoes the review by IRB members who review protocols in the "expedited" category.[3] Even for exempt studies, the IRB opens files, requires annual reports, and for studies involving contacts with subjects (e.g., interviews), often requires researchers to obtain informed consent or to provide subjects with written material including the elements that would appear on a consent form.

---

[3]In the context of HSR, the most relevant exempt category is "research, involving the collection or study of existing data, documents, records, pathological specimens, or diagnostic specimens, if these sources are publicly available or if the information is recorded by the investigator in such a manner that subjects cannot be identified, directly or through identifiers linked to the subjects" (45 CFR 46.101(b)(4)).

Col. Anderson explained that Army regulations are separate from civilian regulations, but that the Army's regulations on human subjects research closely follow the Common Rule as previously presented by Dr. Puglisi. He explained further that the Army's regulations on the treatment of military research subjects have been expanded (by Title 10 USC 980) to include a ban on waiving informed consent when data collected will include identifying information, unless the research is exempt. Finally, he said that the military criteria for exemption are substantively the same as the civilian criteria as codified in the common rule.

Determining Whether Information Is Identifiable in Assessing Risk of Disclosure

Ms. Khan noted that the UTHSCSA IRB continues to wrestle with how to determine whether data would be identifiable. For projects collecting data from computer databases, it asks the investigator to list all the fields to be collected and to indicate who will actually collect the data, how respect for privacy by any personnel involved will be ensured, and how further dissemination of the information will be prevented (e.g., storing data on computers that are not networked, storing codes identifying individuals separately from data, using passwords and/or key requirements to restrict access both to computers for data storage and to computer housing identifying codes).

Col. Anderson explained that the Army tracks all the records associated with a soldier by Social Security number. In the case of certain types of research such as developing vaccines in preparation for missions to other climates or protection of soldiers from possible biological warfare, the military has adopted special precautions for maintaining confidentiality of the records. Although many of the personal privacy issues of civilian life cannot enter into the military environment (i.e., a soldier's health status must be known to his or her supervisors, and he or she cannot deny them access to it because it determines medical qualification to serve), additional privacy protection has been adopted for soldiers who volunteer as the subjects of biological warfare vaccine research. These additional protection measures were adopted because information about the particular vaccines tested might later be used as a basis for the denial of insurance coverage or other benefits or might be used to refuse issuing a visa in cases where the vaccine record suggested an assignment in a nation unfriendly to the United States. Col. Anderson noted that the use of vaccines, whose *names* are the same as those of highly hazardous organisms associated with biological warfare, does not have any real risks greater than those of ordinary vaccines used for the general public, but the names may be frightening. To shield their privacy, soldiers may opt for separate research medical records, stored apart from regular clinical records, so that records regarding research participation remain confidential and under more restricted access.

Weighing Importance of the Research Relative to Risk

Ms. Khan explained that risk to subjects must be balanced against benefits of the research in HSR, as with any protocol. However, in most of the HSR studies, she continued, the subjects themselves are not likely to receive any direct benefit. Thus, the UTHSCSA IRB's tolerance for risk to the subjects tends to be correspondingly low. The IRB tries to assist investigators in identifying possible disclosure risks, stemming, for instance, from overlooked links between fields or retention of identifying information that could be eliminated without jeopardizing the results of the research. Ms. Khan observed that investigators sometimes retain identifying fields as a matter of convenience and sometimes even do so when there is no need for the information. The IRB can assist by alerting investigators to the possible risks and educating them about how to avoid them.

In the review of the privacy issues in an HSR study, Ms. Khan noted that the UTHSCSA IRB considers all those about whom data would be collected, and whose privacy might therefore be at risk. In some protocols, for instance, the set of subjects regarding whom data will be collected includes not only the patients who received a service, but also the health care providers who delivered the service. In this case, the UTHSCSA IRB is concerned that the privacy of health care providers is protected.

Ensuring That Identifiable Information Is Protected During the Study

Ms. Khan explained that the UTHSCSA IRB requires information at the time of the application detailing how the protocol will protect confidentiality. Upon approval, the IRB instructs the investigators that they may not make any changes to these procedures without prior IRB approval. The IRB requires status reports annually or more often. Ms. Khan also noted that for any protocol involving particularly sensitive data, the IRB requires the investigator to obtain a certificate of confidentiality.[4]

Col. Anderson mentioned that an investigator may request that research records be maintained under special coded identification numbers, with a linkage to the individual's Social Security number. The key linking the study identification number and the Social Security number is then stored separately under extremely limited access.

---

[4]The certificate of confidentiality is described in the Public Health Services Act (§301(d)). It provides protection for research data from subpoena by law enforcement agencies. The investigator applies directly to the appropriate official, which varies depending on the nature of the sensitive data. The types of data that may be eligible for protection include information pertaining to sexual matters, drug use, illegal activity, mental health, or other information that could damage the subject's financial standing, reputation, or could be in some way stigmatizing. See also Wolf and Lo, 1999.

Enforcement of Procedures to Protect Confidentiality

Ms. Khan concluded that IRBs function best when working in a collaborative, educational relationship with the investigators. The UTHSCSA IRB requires periodic status reports on all studies but does not itself audit investigators or otherwise engage in active surveillance to ensure compliance. Indeed, if a compliance assurance role proves necessary, she argued that it would be more effectively carried out by another office so as not to lose the positive relationship with investigators that the IRB has developed.

Regarding Col. Anderson's presentation, committee member Peter Szolovits commended the Army's ability to maintain effective barriers between different parts of the organization so as to keep a file of identifiers for use if necessary but not risk improper disclosure, and asked if such a centralized resource for psuedonymizing data could be used at other institutions. Col. Anderson replied that the centralization of subject data demographics, control of data privacy, and enforcement of procedures to maintain them might be implemented effectively in a military organization but be impracticable or impossible in a civilian setting.

Additional Recommendations by Presenters

Ms. Khan offered several additional recommendations. First, in multisite projects, personally identifiable health information generally ought not to be shared beyond the local investigators. Second, she suggested that studies involving collection of data through telephone interviews, which are frequently used to collect information about services rendered (though not the focus of this workshop), should be carefully reviewed and not necessarily approved if the subject's name and telephone number will be given to a contract research organization to make the calls. Finally, Ms. Khan emphasized that IRBs can and should develop collaborative relationships with other parts of their institutions. As an example, she suggested consulting with university committees that review research for appropriateness and research allocation. She explained that since these bodies tend to be concerned with both costs and legal exposure during research, it is important that they and the IRB coordinate their policies. Coordination both avoids frustrating investigators with inconsistent requirements and builds in more internal support for compliance with the policies.

General Discussion Following Presentations

Committee member Lisa Iezzoni commented that some IRBs either prefer, or believe themselves required, to insist on using exactly the same language on the consent form as would be used for clinical trials. In her experience, the result is that potential participants in a health services research study that may involve a review only of their records are warned about risk of physical injury, possibly including death. Ms. Khan and several IRB administrators and/or chairs replied that their IRBs work to ensure that the language of the consent form reflects the actual risks of the protocol.

Dr. Iezzoni also mentioned that one branch of HSR, qualitative health services research, involves detailed interviews with a small sample of patients and that, in these cases, additional precautions are needed to protect the privacy of the participants. For instance, if the interviews are taped or videotaped, the voices and/or faces may have to be masked.

Finally, a member of the audience, Dr. Joanne Lynne of RAND, urged the committee to be mindful of the plight of very small hospices and other health care providers who wish to carry out quality improvement projects. Such organizations may lack the resources to locate or negotiate with an IRB.

Academic IRB Chairs

Dr. James Kahn, chair of the Committee for Human Research at the University of California in San Francisco (UCSF), presented first, followed by Dr. Robert Amdur of the University of Florida, recently IRB chair at Dartmouth Medical School.

Identifying Specific Studies as HSR

Dr. Kahn said that HSR studies at UCSF are reviewed in the same way as other studies involving human subjects, except that the wording in the informed consent form would be modified to reflect the type of research and would not warn of physical injury. Dr. Kahn commented that if data are to be collected systematically, the project ought to be reviewed by the IRB, since it is reasonably likely that the investigator will publish the results if the findings prove to be of interest.

Dr. Amdur said that the differentiation of health services research from various types of health operations such as internal quality assessment is critical and argued that IRBs ought not to take on the task of protecting privacy in non-research settings. Instead, protection of privacy in a nonresearch setting ought to be addressed in other ways. He was concerned not only about the workload of IRBs but also about placing administrative burdens on quality improvement projects and health care operations. He suggested that the way to distinguish research from other activities is to determine whether the project would be done in the same way if the project directors knew they would not be able to publish or otherwise present the results in an academic forum (Amdur et al., in press). That is, if the project would be done even if the findings could not be published or disseminated, it is not research. He pointed out that the fact of publication alone would not be a sufficient criterion because the results of nonresearch assessments are in fact sometimes published, but that research is always undertaken with a view to contributing to public, general, knowledge.

Determining Which HSR Studies Qualify as Exempt

Dr. Amdur argued that current federal regulations are applicable and appropriate for evaluating health services research. Current regulations already allow waiving of informed consent when risk would be minimal and the project could not reasonably be carried out if informed consent were required. From this perspective, he continued, the problem then resolves again to the need for the IRB to take a rigorous view of what is research and to turn back any proposals that ought, under the regulatory definition of research, to be viewed as a health care operations or QA activity.

Weighing Importance of the Research Relative to Risk

Dr. Amdur commented that for IRBs that are operating according to the Common Rule, the fundamental risk assessment approach is not a new task and the regulatory structure is already, for the most part, in place. He continued that reviewing HSR protocols, in particular the evaluation of risks associated with possible invasions of privacy or breaches of confidentiality, does not make the risk assessment task any different. An IRB could need additional knowledge or expertise about how privacy might be invaded (whether intentionally or inadvertently) since some means now available have only recently been developed.

Additional Recommendations by Presenters

Dr. Kahn reported that in response to several recent incidents in which the IRBs of other institutions had been criticized for inadequate oversight, the vice chancellor of the UCSF had commissioned an ad hoc committee to consider some specific questions in reviewing the UCSF IRB's function. The ad hoc committee was asked to consider the composition, procedures, and support of the IRB and whether it could be of better service to the university. The committee returned a list of recommendations, including several suggestions about increasing the use of electronic information systems, increased training for researchers to address both research responsibilities and institutional procedures, and increasing staff support for the human subjects protection program. In addition, the chair specifically suggested designating 1 to 1.5 percent of each grant involving human subjects to be earmarked as funding for the human subjects protection program.

Dr. Amdur suggested that the growth of multisite research projects would require changes in IRB function and structure. Because many HSR projects depend on data from many different sites, the current system of review by each local IRB creates an administrative burden that may discourage valuable HSR projects. He suggested testing a central IRB to review multisite HSR studies.

General Discussion Following Presentations

In additional general discussion, committee member Lisa Iezzoni mentioned experiences where different IRBs from different institutions are involved and return inconsistent assessments. Several participants agreed that this is not uncommon and must be resolved by negotiation on a case-by-case basis.

In discussions of problems turning on what party has a claim to data, either for gaining or for withholding access, several participants asked to whom the data belonged. Committee member Adele Waller explained that, as a legal matter, disputes over how to handle data between different institutions cannot be resolved simply by determining ownership of the data. She continued that several parties typically have legitimate rights and responsibilities pertaining to the data, distinctions that the concept "ownership" is unable to capture, and that no single party has ownership.

Research Institute IRB Chairs

Research institutes that are separate from universities carry out a great deal of HSR. When such research is federally funded, these institutions are subject to the Common Rule. Some research institutes have multiple project assurances [5] through the OPRR in which they have agreed to comply with the Common Rule for any human subjects research. The research institutes that participated in the workshop are not affiliated with health care organizations such as integrated health care systems or health maintenance organizations (HMOs), so they do not face the issue of distinguishing HSR from quality improvement or business functions. Because research institutes do not carry out clinical care or payment, all of their activities would be research.

The first presenter was Dr. Tora Bikson, senior social scientist and IRB chair at RAND. She was followed by Dr. Steven A. Garfinkel, an IRB chair and health services researcher at Research Triangle Institute (RTI).

RAND's multiple project assurance agreement stipulates that the institution will be guided by the ethical principles in the Belmont Report (Belmont, 1979) and will adhere to federal regulations regarding human subjects protection for all research involving human subjects regardless of sponsorship. RTI also follows the Common Rule in all human subjects research.

Identifying Specific Studies as HSR

Dr. Bikson noted that the organizational unit that carries out a study cannot be viewed as an indication of whether the study is HSR. Various parts of

---

[5]An "assurance" is an agreement or contract between an institution and the OPRR, on behalf of the Secretary of Health and Human Services. The assurance stipulates the methods by which the institution will protect the welfare of research subjects in accordance with the regulations. An MPA is a type of assurance designed for institutions that engage in large amounts of health-related research. An MPA can be approved for 5-year intervals.

RAND, including the health research program, but also for example, the education program and the criminal justice program, carry out HSR studies but they are reviewed by the same IRB. As noted above, RAND requires all its research involving human subjects to be in accord with the common rule and to be reviewed by its IRB.

Dr. Garfinkel said that RTI does surveillance, cost and use studies (for example, an evaluation of Oregon's Medicaid Reform Project), program evaluation, and outcomes assessments. RTI also does coordination of clinical trials and epidemiological work. In the former areas, it works with medical records and insurance enrollment and claims (as well as interviews and tissue specimens). RTI actually maintains three IRBs, two of which include physicians. The HSR proposals go to the third IRB, which does not include physicians, for review.

Determining Which HSR Qualify Studies as Exempt

The committee heard that RAND has implemented an on-line system to ensure that there is appropriate IRB review of all protocols. The IRB is notified whenever a project receives an internal funding account number—in fact, assigning such a number automatically triggers a message to the investigator containing a brief screening questionnaire about the project. If the screener indicates that the project might require IRB review, a more detailed questionnaire then helps the investigator explore alternatives of exemption from IRB review, expedited review, or full review (Figure 2-2). The on-line system may indicate that a project would be exempt from IRB review if it will use only anonymous or public use datasets or de-identified data sets if neither RAND nor any another party on the contract has access to the identifiers. Dr. Bikson emphasized that the system is designed to be inclusive, that is, to send any borderline cases to IRB members for specific attention. In less clear situations, the IRB chair and/or selected members would have to decide whether the particular project could be exempt. Examples of borderline situations where an IRB member would have to examine the project to decide whether further IRB review might be needed include projects that will use anonymous or nonsensitive primary data gathered through surveys, interviews or other methods requiring a direct interaction with subjects; projects that gather data from public officials or candidates; or intervention research that is anonymous and without risk.

Determining Whether Information Is Identifiable in
Assessing Risk of Disclosure

Dr. Bikson noted that the determination of whether identifiable information will be involved remains challenging, and it is important to realize that identifiability could enter the process at various points, from subject selection to data combination to subject compensation. She reminded participants that information may be directly identifiable (e.g., a Social Security number) but may also be

134

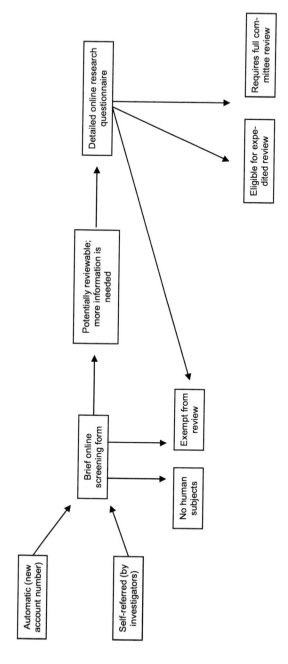

FIGURE 2-2 RAND's system for identifying reviewable research. SOURCE: Adapted from slide presented by Dr. Tora Bikson at the Workshop on Institutional Review Boards and Health Services Research Data Privacy.

identifiable by inference from the combination of several data fields—identifiability by inference is therefore one of the key concerns of privacy in research utilizing databases. She suggested a general rule used by RAND that may be of interest to others: if sorting data according to any variables produces subsets with ten or fewer members, then these individuals will be at risk for identifiability by inference.

Dr. Bikson, seconded by several participants, commented that researchers often would strongly prefer to work with de-identified data, but that even if they request such data and supply de-identifying algorithms to providers, they may receive data complete with identifiers because the provider lacked time and staff to remove identifying fields.

Dr. Garfinkel commented that when RTI researchers collect data from surveys and claims, they are often required to produce public use files as part of the product. He noted that in the course of producing such files, they have likewise had to work at the problem of determining which fields may lead to identifiability or at least increase the risk of unintended disclosure of personal information.

Weighing Importance of the Research Relative to Risk

Dr. Garfinkel explained that when RTI plans to produce a public access file, it informs respondents that their data will be kept confidential, by which it means that data will not be released in an identifiable form. He reported that in RTI's experience, informing respondents that their data will be included in a public use file, even though not in identifiable form, will needlessly lower the response rate. He observed that the scientific benefit of a study could be seriously impaired by unnecessarily alarming individuals about their privacy in the consent form.

Ensuring That Identifiable Information Is Protected During the Study

Dr. Bikson said that RAND's IRB includes a three-person privacy team. The team, includes an information resource specialist (who specializes in security measures such as encryption and creating codes to substitute for identifying data), a data librarian (who specializes in rules and practices for dealing with very large datasets acquired from other organizations), and a network specialist (who specializes in conditions and limitations of safe data transfer over the network). These IRB members help design and implement data safeguarding plans commensurate with the level of risk for various protocols. Dr. Bikson emphasized that data safeguarding includes maintaining physical control of the data especially while in transit and that the risk of physical access to data by unauthorized parties is sometimes overlooked even while more sophisticated technical security measures may be attended to.

Beyond physical delivery, Dr. Bikson continued, the treatment of datasets to be merged and manipulated is important to preserve data integrity and also to protect subject privacy. RAND's suggested procedure calls for first replacing any direct identifiers with codes. The file linking the code to the subject's identity is then encrypted and stored separately from the encoded data file. Then when another dataset is obtained, it is possible to regenerate the link file, replace direct identifiers in the new file with the subject codes, and merge the coded files.

Dr. Bikson noted that because physical and technical protections are not sufficient, RAND has implemented procedural protective measures. These procedures include annual reviews for all projects, including inactive projects, until such time as the direct identifiers and link files have been destroyed and any remaining data that might be identifiable by inference have been eliminated or altered so that identities cannot be inferred.

Dr. Garfinkel discussed briefly some situations in which beneficence may require breach of confidentiality. RTI would consider such a breach in cases of subjects exhibiting suicidal ideation or intent. Child abuse is another difficult area, and the reporting of cases may be required in some states. Dr. Garfinkel described an RTI project on child abuse in which researchers review records from county social services with varying reporting laws. Since the laws differ by locale, RTI designed a uniform national guideline and consent form and then asked local interviewers to inform RTI when they were in danger of differing from local laws.

Dr. Garfinkel said that in some studies they receive coded data, for example, Medicare enrollment data with ID codes but no names or addresses, so the investigators can track costs and utilization by each subject without knowing the identity of these individuals. In other instances, Dr. Garfinkel noted, they might receive files of names and addresses for the purpose of contacting individuals. When they make a contact, they first ask permission from the individual to continue the project and to do a data linkage, thus obtaining an "ex post facto" consent (or dropping the individual from the study if this is what the individual prefers).

Enforcement of Procedures to Protect Confidentiality

Dr. Bikson said that RAND has observed that networked, distributed, and backed-up digital environments together pose new types of threats to privacy. Some researchers, for instance, may not realize that taking a diskette with backup files home to work on a personal computer that is connected to a Digital Subscriber Line (DSL) line (which is on all the time) can create a serious security breach. Such examples suggest that the role of technical experts may be underappreciated, and new technologies to protect privacy may yet be unexplored or insufficiently exploited. She concluded that policy control must be developed to replace physical oversight to ensure privacy protection, because it is in many cases impossible, and surely impractical, to observe directly whether researchers carrying out electronic manipulations are conforming to data protection rules.

Additional Recommendations by Presenters

Dr. Bikson observed that professionals in other areas of study already have gained long experience in the types of privacy concerns that HSR is now facing, so researchers in health services might learn from, for example, researchers in the criminal justice system.

Dr. Garfinkel reaffirmed the importance of health services researchers' having the freedom to work with their IRBs to modify standard consent and confidentiality language as appropriate for the particular study in question.

Dr. Garfinkel also commented on the distinct issue of studies using tissue specimens (although not the primary focus of this project), saying that requirements for informed consent for tissue storage are as yet misunderstood by some researchers. In addition, such research raises issues of how to communicate storage provisions on the consent form. The consent form separates stages of consent, requesting the candidate to consider and consent separately to participation in the study, to provision of the specimen, and then to allowing the specimen to be stored for later use.

Commercial, Nonaffiliated IRBs

Although the traditional model of an IRB envisions a board closely associated with a particular institution that draws its membership from the institution and surrounding community, there are also nonaffiliated or freestanding IRBs that provide review services for a fee. For many, the bulk of their business involves clinical trials, but some also review health services research. Some nonaffiliated IRBs regard their niche as providing consultative services primarily to relatively small institutions that do not have MPAs and therefore might find the support of an in-house IRB review to be difficult. Dr. Angela Bowen, chief executive officer of Western Institutional Review Board (WIRB) attended the workshop and spoke about WIRB.

Determining Which HSR Studies Qualify as Exempt

A central feature of WIRB's approach is its commitment to making individual, specific, informed consent a part of all human subjects research it sees.

Several health services researchers pointed out that since it is not uncommon for HSR protocols to utilize databases containing on the order of hundreds of thousands or even millions of records, it would be difficult to design a workable individual informed consent associated with a particular research protocol. Dr. Bowen replied, however, that protocols of this type rarely, if ever, go to commercial IRBs, so WIRB has not experienced that particular problem.

*Determining Whether Information Is Identifiable in
Assessing Risk of Disclosure*

Like other IRBs, the WIRB committee struggles with determining whether data will be identifiable. In reviewing protocols for potential privacy risks, it considers data to be identifiable if there is any link between the data and the subject's identity, in which case, again, it would insist on informed consent by the subject.

General Discussion Following Presentation

Several participants raised questions about how nonaffiliated IRBs can take into account the values and attitudes of the community in which the research is conducted. Dr. Bowen explained that nonaffiliated IRBs can develop solid relationships with clients, especially repeat clients, so they work closely with the local institutions. Other discussion addressed the accountability of a nonaffiliated IRB, since it does not report directly to an institution, and Dr. Bowen noted that commercial IRBs are audited regularly by the FDA and OPRR.

HEALTH CARE PRODUCTS AND
SERVICES INDUSTRY

Many health care organizations carry out a spectrum of activities that involve the secondary analysis of personal health information. The spectrum ranges from health services research to operations. Representatives of several types of organizations that are largely concerned with the delivery of health services—that is, operations—along with research functions spoke about their experience in the review of HSR by IRBs.

Pharmaceutical Manufacturer's Epidemiological Research

Dr. Harry Guess, executive director of epidemiology at Merck Research Laboratories, discussed epidemiological surveillance of drugs and vaccines as carried out within a pharmaceutical company. The purpose of these studies is to assess the efficacy and safety of the product in clinical trials and the safety of the product in actual postmarketing use. Much of the epidemiological analysis utilizes previously collected data.

Identifying Specific Studies as Research under the Regulations

Dr. Guess explained that in most cases, although not federally funded, pharmaceutical company epidemiological work will be under the purview of the Common Rule, either because it is subject to regulation by the Food and Drug Administration or because it is done in conjunction with a university or other organization that requires it.

Ensuring That Identifiable Information Is Protected During the Study

Dr. Guess observed that the approaches used to protect confidentiality of data in research sponsored by pharmaceutical companies differ by type of data. In the case of adverse event reporting, he explained, the company may be unable to avoid knowing the identity of the patient or the physician because one of these individuals actually called in the report. Such information is subject to additional levels of security. The reports to regulatory agencies do not identify patients or physicians. In clinical trials, however, he said that the identity of the participants is generally not given to the Merck officials at all, but rather is replaced by a code at each study site. For protection of privacy, he concluded, Merck must therefore rely on the IRBs and investigators at each study site, since the identifiable information generally is not transmitted to Merck. He continued that for other potentially identifying information, such as birthdates, Merck typically requests that only ranges be reported whenever possible. Finally, Dr. Guess noted that Merck audits study sites to make sure they are in compliance with FDA regulations and the FDA also conducts inspections.

Enforcement of Procedures to Protect Confidentiality

The situation of records research at Merck was of particular interest at the workshop because of the affiliation of Merck with Medco, a pharmacy benefit management company. In the discussion after the presentation, participants inquired about the degree of separation between the Merck research databases and the Medco administrative and pharmacy usage databases. Dr. Guess said that federal trade law requires the two branches of the company to be unambiguously separate with regard to inside information. Thus, when other divisions of Merck wish to utilize data from Merck-Medco for research, they must negotiate a purchase of access to the data as any other research organization would.

Intermountain Health Care

Intermountain Health Care is a not-for-profit integrated health care delivery system, including hospitals and clinics in four states and tertiary services in a larger area. The organization has strongly promoted electronic medical records since the 1950s. Dr. Brent James and Mr. Morris Linton of Intermountain Health Care participated in the workshop.

Identifying Specific Studies as HSR

Dr. James began with the persistent problem of distinguishing the activities of HSR from operations, since Intermountain Health Care (IHC), unlike the research foundations, does both. He explained that IHC views these activities as encompassing a continuum ranging from health care operations performance assessment, to records review or epidemiological research, to clinical research. Then, in this view, confidentiality protection also forms a continuum (Figure 2-3).

Dr. James said that the clinical research end of the spectrum is overseen by an IRB, and confidentiality concerns pertaining to clinical research would also be reviewed by the IRB. The hospitals in the IHC system that do the most research have an MPA and shared IRB structure. Investigations and analyses on the health care operations end of the spectrum that do not meet the definition of "research," do not fall under the purview of IRB oversight. Here Dr. James observed that when IRBs go beyond their original role of protecting human subjects from direct harms due to research, they may tend both to cause confusion and to neglect their primary mission. Finally, Dr. James noted that just as the vast majority of uses of patient data occur in the course of health care operations, so also the vast majority of breaches of confidentiality occur in operations (indeed he said that all the known privacy violations in IHC have occurred in health care operations, none in research).

Determining Which HSR Studies Qualify as Exempt

Dr. James explained that IHC has an Information Security Committee, which it believes may be similar to the privacy boards described in the proposed rule. This committee is constituted similarly to an IRB, consisting of community members as well as line administrators and scientists (including computer specialists). The committee oversees and coordinates IRB functions in the organization. It also determines whether projects from the area in the middle of the health care operations and research spectrum should proceed to seek IRB review.

Ensuring That Identifiable Information Is Protected During the Study

Dr. James continued that the Information Security Committee generates and recommends data security policies to the Board of Trustees of the company. The committee then helps implement the policies and procedures throughout the organization.

Enforcement of Procedures to Protect Confidentiality

Dr. James said that, first, all IHC employees must sign a confidentiality agreement, which must be renewed every two years, and then comply with a "need-to-know" policy limiting who has access to which data. The company also tracks data access with automatic electronic logs and has designed the elec- tronic records system to ensure that identifiable portions are accessible only to designated employees. IHC terminates employment because of privacy infractions.

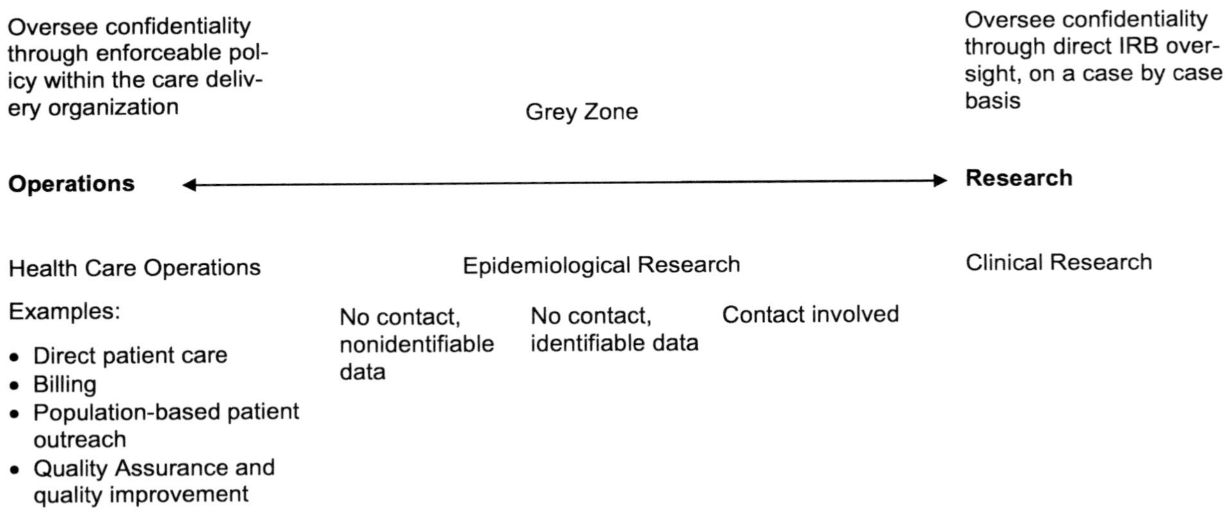

FIGURE 2-3 Intermountain Health Care's approach to operations: research spectrum. SOURCE: adapted from a slide presented by Dr. Brent James at the Workshop on Institutional Review Boards and Health Services Research Data Privacy.

Dr. James expects the user authentication problem to be addressed much more effectively in the future with, for instance, biological log-ons[1] rather than passwords to restrict access.

Additional Recommendations by Presenter

Dr. James noted that IHC believes that patients as well as providers should be able to view their own records and add comments (although nothing can be changed or deleted). With rare exceptions, IHC-covered patients have this access.

Regarding patient perception of privacy, Dr. James observed that many types of professionals within a health system generate and use patient information and that patients understand that many professionals, as well their own physicians, will need access to their medical records. It is important to be sensitive to patients' perceptions, however, so when it is necessary to contact the patient for a research project or other purposes, the contact should be initiated by a professional who would be, and would be perceived by the patient as being, reasonably expected to have access to the patient's records.

Finally, Dr. James suggested that truly de-identifying a health care record is impossible if there is any link to any potentially identifying information. Hence, the way to minimize confidentiality breaches is to control access to the link that leads to identifiability. He suggested further that a record is identified only when a human being sees it, so that if a computer program links records using identifiable data but returns a nonidentifiable output, then that would not constitute a privacy violation.

Pharmacy Benefit Management Company

Ms. Jennifer Low and Dr. Fred Teitelbaum of Express Scripts discussed privacy and confidentiality in the context of pharmacy benefit management. Express Scripts is a pharmacy benefit management (PBM) company, serving various types of clients including insurers, unions, health care organizations, and employers—any type of organization, in short, that wishes to contract for a

---

[1]Biological log-ons, also called biometric identifiers, would permit a user to have access to a file based on some recognizable and unique feature. In Wiederhold's on-line glossary, (http://www-db.stanford.edu/pub/gio/CS99I/security.html#BIOMETRIC) biometric identifiers are explained as follows: are more reliable than passwords. Biometric identifiers: voice prints, signature dynamics, keystroke dynamics, hand measurements, finger prints, face recognition. The pattern of the iris in a person's eye is also a candidate for making a unique identification. Biometric identifiers are difficult to forge, but the equipment needed to read them is awkward and forbidding. The person being identified must cooperate for instance be willing to speak or write a specific expression clearly or be scanned by a camera in a well-lighted space. Voice recognition is probably the easiest technique to integrate into computer workstations. The voice pattern can also be recorded on a smartcard, which can be linked securely to its owner. That card can contain passwords, that are easily handled by the networks that verify access privileges.

pharmacy benefit. Among other things, the company provides pharmacy network management, claim adjudication services, and drug utilization review and also functions as a mail service pharmacy.

Identifying Specific Studies as HSR

Ms. Low and Dr. Teitelbaum both observed that, as members of a PBM company, it is difficult if not impossible for them to distinguish HSR from operations. Express Scripts conducts internal analyses of data to improve operations (e.g., plan design, but also formulary decisions and assessment of outcomes), although results are published whenever possible. However, confidentiality standards (which include the protection and ultimate purging of identifiable data) apply when such data are first used to create the research data set.

Ms. Low explained that, especially when it was smaller, the company regarded itself as a pharmacy and thus bound by professional standards and law without need for additional policy. As the size and scope of its operations increased, the company has undertaken more formal policy development. She also said that the company's primary means of ensuring that its appropriate authorization to use data on patients is by asking the plan sponsor (i.e., the managed care organization, employer, etc.) to obtain authorization from individual plan participants.

Determining Whether Information Is Identifiable in Assessing Risk of Disclosure

Dr. Teitelbaum reported that Express Scripts has instituted increasingly stringent policies of limiting internal access to data.

Ensuring That Identifiable Information Is Protected During the Study

Dr. Teitelbaum described processes of data use: the data are typically kept in a de-identified format, with a cross-reference for identification stored separately and securely. De-identification of the data includes not only the removal of names but also, for example, the use of age rather than date of birth and the use of only the first three digits of the zip code.

Dr. Teitelbaum continued that the company is in the process of instituting a privacy board to ensure that it does follow appropriate and effective procedures for maintaining confidentiality. Its practices regarding data retention vary according to state law (typically two to three years for prescriptions) or Employee Retirement Income Security Act (ERISA) (six to seven years), but de-identified data may be kept indefinitely.

Health Maintenance Organizations and Research

Mr. Andrew Nelson, executive director of HealthPartners and president of the HMO Research Network, offered some perspective on the amount of HSR that occurs in the managed care industry.

Mr. Nelson reported that the fraction of HMOs that formally and regularly engage in research is relatively small (Nelson et al., 1998). There are 1,315 licensed managed care organizations, 24 of which have formal research programs doing public domain research. Of the 24 HMOs that are active in research 13 established the HMO Research Network. Mr. Nelson also noted that many of these HMO-based research organizations follow the Common Rule whether the funding source would require it or not.

Mr. Nelson said that, like many observers, he has noted that many IRBs are busy to the point of being overwhelmed and that increasing demands on them also decrease the satisfaction of what is, in many cases, voluntary work. He offered for consideration ten recommendations to help ease the overall problem of properly protecting confidentiality in HSR without unduly stressing IRBs. The first six address recommendations what institutions need; the last four are external to the research HMO:

1. A framework to define the intersection between research and quality improvement.

2. An internal auditing process.

3. Training and educational programs.

4. Individual data access and confidentiality certification for anyone who may have access.

5. Internal and external data access policy as a broad foundation for data privacy.

6. Information technology policy defining how to apply privacy protections.

7. Encouraging academic institutions to incorporate research ethics and research subjects protections into their curricula,

8. Development ready-to-use tools for HSR investigators to apply.

9. Asking IRBs to apply the Common Rule regardless of the funding source of the study.

10. Increasing government involvement to include education as well as oversight of IRBs.

SPECIAL CONSIDERATIONS OF DATA PRIVACY AND MINORITY GROUPS

Dr. William Freeman, IRB chair at the Indian Health Service, highlighted some issues of particular importance in research involving minority populations. He concentrated on American Indian, Alaska Native, Canadian First Nations,

Inuit, and Kanaka Maoli or Native Hawaiian groups. Dr. Freeman emphasized that he has not seen any specific instance of harm to minority groups due to HSR, but the potential for privacy violation exists. He noted further that the potential harm may affect not only the individuals and groups that might be subjects, but also the research enterprise because if a group participates in research and regards the privacy of the group or individual members to have been violated, then any researcher approaching that group or perhaps other groups, as well, will not be able to secure cooperation.

Levels of Privacy Concerns

Dr. Freeman pointed out that HSR usually addresses large sets of data in which individual subjects may have little in common and are difficult to identify. He suggested that in local, small, minority groups the situation is quite different, with serious implications for privacy. First, he noted, the groups mentioned are often relatively small and isolated communities whose members are well known to one another, so the privacy of individuals within the group may be much more difficult to protect than the privacy of an individual in a large city with a diverse population. At the same time, a second type of privacy concern can affect such populations. Because the minority group in question may have strong intracommunity ties and be distinct from the surrounding culture or cultures in significant respects, its members are likely to place a high value on the integrity of the group. In this context, privacy may refer to the group as a whole rather than to individuals.

Strategies for Enhancing Both Privacy Protection and Trust

Dr. Freeman reaffirmed that both physical and electronic data security are very important and frequently not given adequate attention in rural areas. He also pointed out that data fields that might appear at first sight not to be identifying in a large population could lead to the identification of one or a few individuals in a small community. He suggested that the way to avoid such mistakes would be to include in the protocol review, consultation with individuals knowledgeable about the particular culture or group in question. He also suggested that in some cases the use of formal, individual contracts—in which the researchers promise not to attempt to identify any individual and to notify the IRB if an individual may have been identified inadvertently—may help build the trust of the community in the research project.

General Discussion

In the discussion after the presentation, several participants raised the questions of what is an appropriate role for the community in the research process and of how to involve affected parties in the community when there is no cohesive group and therefore no generally accepted spokesperson (though many, of course volunteering for that role, with divergent views). Although a definitive answer did not emerge, several participants suggested that it is generally possible to speak with several groups when there is no single representative.

TECHNICAL CONSIDERATIONS AND PRODUCTS

Mr. Lawrence Dietz of AXENT Technologies, an attorney and market research analyst specializing in information security, briefed the committee on market and technical trends in data security.

Web access security products are becoming increasingly necessary for security maintenance and enhancement as more organizations wish to store, retrieve, and exchange information via intranet. Although the products are emerging, it is not yet clear what the costs may be of providing full servicing for them.

Regarding public key infrastructure (PKI), the industry and researchers are very enthusiastic, and some observers believe the HIPAA and several laws in the European Union to be driving the market to develop PKI products.[2] Market adoption of PKI is, however, proceeding only slowly, especially in the United States. This may be due at least in part to the fact that the process of integrating PKI with individual legacy applications is very labor intensive. One reason integration is difficult is that it is so complex; indeed, a PKI encryption device may be asked to solve a wide variety of problems including authentication, access, and authorization. The development and market penetration of smart cards and other portable platforms for utilizing databases via PKI seems to be much further advanced in Europe than in the United States, although unresolved questions about cross-border privacy protection remain.

As the technology of Web-integrated systems becomes more ubiquitous and easier to use, it is also becoming more difficult to defend from outside attack (Dietz, 2000). Internal and external filtering techniques can be viewed as necessary in any operation utilizing electronic records, since it would be critical to minimize any time when the system is not available. Filtering systems, for example, would be able to detect a pattern when a denial-of-service attack is launched from multiple points requesting the same data at the same time and also can guard against local systems being co-opted from the outside to serve as launching points for such an attack (also described as "being used as zombies").

---

[2]A public key infrastructure is a system for managing and distributing public keys and digital certificates to authenticate different users—that is, to ensure that the asserted identity of a given user in fact corresponds to user. (In face-to-face interactions, one person can "authenticate" himself to another by presenting a document such as a driver's license or a passport. By telephone, a speaker can authenticate himself to another person by virtue of a familiar voice. In cyberspace, however, some other mechanism is needed to provide authentication among parties that do not know in advance that they need to interact—that mechanism is PKI.) PKIs are an essential component of secure electronic communications, but also raise important concerns for privacy (see for example, Brands, 1999).

Cost pressures are of course resulting in both specific and general trends. Specifically, many or perhaps most organizations are installing virtual private networks, enhancing security relative to standard internet e-mail while also saving money. More generally, many organizations are exhibiting a marked preference to hire services, that is, to contract out to meet their information technology needs, rather than to purchase products and train in-house support; this practice has corresponding security risks as more people have access to electronic records while being less invested in the culture of the organization.

In the future, additional work on security will likely be required at the small office and home office level, a point that often arises in consideration of academic researchers who deal with secure data but often work at home.

SPECIAL CONSIDERATIONS OF DATA PRIVACY AND MINORS[3]

Federal regulations on human subjects include special provisions that apply when subjects are of minor age (45 CFR 46 Subpart D). The contract describing the IOM's project included an agreement that the committee would consider measures for protecting personally identifiable health information that pertains to children if any different conditions should be deemed desirable, and, in particular, would consider the desirability of requiring projects involving children always to undergo full IRB review. For background on these matters, the committee commissioned a paper on protecting the data from health services research in minors. The paper was presented in draft form at the workshop and appears in full as appendix C of the (IOM, 2000) report.

There are three basic issues that further complicate the question of how to conduct research involving minors that meets high ethical and scientific standards:

- the heterogeneity of the population in question,
- complications arising from proxy consent, and
- the changing interests and risks affecting the subjects.

The heterogeneity of the subject population arises from the intersection of the legal definition of the term "minor" with the developmental process of maturation from infancy to adulthood. The law recognizes any person under the age of majority, for most purposes 18 years old, as a child, but the maturation of a person from infancy through the age of majority is a dynamic process, encompassing a very wide range of capacities, interests, concerns, and also risks.

The law recognizes that children do not have the decision-making capacity of adults and addresses this fact through beneficent paternalism. In the case of medical or research interventions, beneficent paternalism requires that consent for the intervention be made by an adult proxy, in most cases the child's par-

---

[3]This section is based on a presentation by Dr. Ross Thompson, developmental psychologist and author of the commissioned paper author.

ent(s). The question of uncoerced and informed consent to participate in research brings with it problems when subjects are adults, and proxy consent brings further complications. In some cases, the adult proxy may have interests that differ from, or even conflict with, those of the child. A further complication arises when the child does reach the age of majority: if an adult has given proxy consent for data on the child to be examined in research, is this consent still valid when the child reaches adulthood, or must consent be sought anew?

The maturation of children not only means that the category "children" is heterogeneous, as described above, but also that as a particular individual matures, the interests of this individual change and the changes themselves are complex. The law—and most people—readily recognize that research on children involves special risks, which must be taken into account and do not apply to adult subjects. The risks, concerns and areas of vulnerability of children do not, however, necessarily diminish inversely with an increase in age and body mass; indeed, some risks increase. Risks that may increase as the child matures include vulnerability to embarrassment, fear of exposure, and concern for violations of privacy—just the risks most likely to be associated with health services research.

In the discussion after the presentation, participants raised several additional points. In consideration of protecting privacy, some features of children as subjects increase the difficulty of de-identifying data. For example, hospitalization is rare for children, so even within a large sample of children, data on hospitalization or very high medical bills may effectively identify one or a small number of individuals. Another special problem is that the effect of the identification of individual children might have additional impact on other family members, since the mother may then be identified as well.

Participant Gerald S. Schatz pointed out that the difficulties associated with proxy consent are further intensified in the case of children who are wards of the state, and proxies who are government agencies and liable to be overburdened or to prefer not to see problems.

INTERNATIONAL COMPARISONS OF DATA PRIVACY STANDARDS[4]

Questions and issues of protecting privacy and personally identifiable health information have arisen in nation states around the world and in regard to the transfer of data across international borders. The contract describing the IOM's project included an agreement that the committee would compare the privacy protections contained in international conventions for personally identifiable health information used in research with the principles and best practices developed in this study. For background on these matters, the committee commissioned a paper comparing international approaches to protecting the privacy of

---

[4]This section is based on a presentation by Ms. Bartha Maria Knoppers, professor of international law.

data from health services research. The paper was presented in draft form at the workshop and appears in full as appendix D of (IOM, 2000) report.

The Organization for Economic cooperation and Development (OECD) published Guidelines on the Protection of Privacy and Transborder Flows of Information in 1989, which included eight basic principles on the collection, use, and holding of personal data; these are further distilled here into four core principles pertaining to data protection, including the creation of statutory protections, transparency of data processing, additional protections for sensitive data, and the rights of individuals to claim enforcement of rules on data protection. The concept of privacy and the principle that individuals ought to be secure from improper interference in privacy are also mentioned in other international agreements including the United Nations *Universal Declaration* (1948) and *International Covenant on Civil and Political Rights* (1966); the European Convention on Human Rights (1955); the Council of Europe's *Convention for the Protection of Individuals, with Regard to Automatic Processing of Data* (1981), *Convention on Human Rights and Biomedicine* (1997), and subsequent recommendations; the World Health Organization's *Declaration on the Promotion of Patient's Rights in Europe* (1994) and *Directive on the Protection of Individuals* (1995); the World Medical Association's *Revised Declaration of Lisbon on the Rights of the Patient* (1995); and the European Group on Ethics in Science and New Technologies' *Ethical Issues of Health Care in the Information Society* (1999).

Turning to the internal or domestic arrangements in selected nation states, the United Kingdom and other Common Law countries such as Australia and New Zealand recognize the protection of privacy under Common Law, although the law can be modified or clarified by statute. Privacy under the Common Law is an aspect of the liberty of a citizen, and if this liberty is infringed upon so as to cause harm, the citizen can pursue legal action. As an exception to the general protection of privacy, however, a medical practitioner may be required to disclose certain information in court if called for by the public interest. Australia also follows Common Law with some statutory exceptions, one of which provides that medical records are considered the property of the private medical practitioner, but not of the public health facility.

By contrast, the legal systems of continental nation states did not develop under Common Law, but follow the Napoleonic Code and variations. Rather than being an aspect of liberty that might be harmed, privacy in this system is viewed as a right in and of itself, which means that a citizen need not show that an infringement of privacy caused harm—an infringement of privacy is sufficient for legal action regardless of whether harm followed. In France, the confidentiality of medical records is further protected by being treated as an obligation of result, which means that not only what is heard or seen is protected by law, but also what is understood, and the body of law that protects the information from disclosure is the penal code.

In the domestic legal systems of individual nation states, the Common Law versus civil code contrast is again the basic distinction. The United Kingdom's British Medial Association has recently affirmed that any disclosure should be anonymous and minimized to the degree possible and that patients should be informed of how data about them may be used. Australian law includes several sets of principles and guidelines, that call for the entity in possession of a record containing personal information to use the information only for the purpose for which it had been collected unless either the subject consents or another use is mandated by other law. France has recently undergone two important developments pertaining to the protection of the privacy of health information in its legal system. The first was a statute regulating the use of data for research, that provided significant new oversight mechanisms, and second was a decree regarding the use of data in the process of reimbursement.

At the conclusion of the presentations, the committee again thanked all the participants for their effort to provide information and insight, and encouraged anyone wishing to comment further or submit written materials to feel free to do so through the study director.

References

Amdur, Robert, Speers, Marjorie A., and Bankert, Elizabeth. IRB Triage of Projects that Involve Medical Record Review. In press.

Applebaum, Paul S. Threats to the Confidentiality of Medical Records—No Place to Hide. JAMA. 2000 Feb 9; 283(6):795–796.

Association of American Medical Colleges. AAMC Comments on The Recommendations of the Secretary of Health and Human Services on the "Confidentiality of Individually Identifiable Health Information." AAMC Testimony Presented to the Senate Labor and Human Resources Committee. 1997 Nov 10.

Belmont 1979. The Belmont Report. Office of the Secretary. Ethical Principles and Guidelines for the Protection of Human Subjects of Research. The National Commission for the Protection of Human Subjects of Biomedical and Behavioral Research. 1979 April.

Bradburn, Norman M. Population—Based Survey Research. Presentation Done at National Bioethics Advisory Commission. 2000 Apr 6.

Brands, Stefan. Rethinking public key infrastructures and digital certificates—building in privacy. Thesis of Stefan Brands. 1999 Sep 4:304 pages.

Buckovich, Suzy A., Rippen, Helga E., and Rozen, Michael J. Driving Toward Guiding Principles: A Goal for Privacy, Confidentiality, and Security of Health Information. Journal of American Medical Informatics Association. 1999 Mar–1999 Apr 30; 6(2):123–133.

Department of Health and Human Services, and Office of the Secretary. Standards for Privacy of Individually Identifiable Health Information; Proposed Rule. Federal Register. 1999 Nov 3; 64(212):59918.

Dietz, Lawrence. Information Warfare Poses New Threats: Are You Ready? Internet Security Advisor. 2000 Mar–2000 Apr. 30:8–10.

Etzioni, Amitai. Medical Records. Enhancing Privacy, Preserving the Common Good. Hastings Center Report. 1999 Mar–1999 Apr 30:14–23.

GHPP (Health Privacy Working Group). Best Principles for Health Privacy. Health Privacy Project; Institute for Health Care Research and Policy, Georgetown University.1999. Available [online] http://www.healthprivacy.org/latest/Best_Principles_Report.pdf.

Goldman, Janlori, and Hudson, Zoe. A Health Privacy Primer for Consumers EXPOSED. Health Privacy Project. Institute for Health Care Research and Policy. Georgetown University. Washington, DC. 1999 Dec. Available [online] http://www.healthprivacy.org/resources/exposed.pdf.

Gostin, Lawrence O., Lazzarini, Zita; Neslund, Verla, and Osterholm, Michael T. The Public Health Information Infrastructure A National Review of the Law on Health Information Privacy. JAMA. 1996 Jun 26; 275(24):1921–1927.

IOM (Institute of Medicine). Committee on Regional Health Data Networks and Molla Donaldson, and Kathleen N. Lohr, editors. Health Data in the Information Age: Use, Disclosure, and Privacy. 1994. Washington, DC: National Academy Press.

IOM (Institute of Medicine). Committee on Health Services Research: Training and Work Force Issues and Marilyn J. Field, Robert E. Tranquada and Jill C. Feasley, editors. Health Services Research: Work. Washington, DC: National Academy Press. 1995.

IOM (Institute of Medicine) Committee on the Role of Institutional Review Boards in Health Services Research Data Privacy Protection. *Protecting Data Privacy in Health Services Research.* Forthcoming. Washington, DC: National Academy Press.

ISPE (International Society for Pharmacoepidemiology). Data privacy, medical record confidentiality, and research in the interest of public health. [Web Page]. 1997 Sep 1. Available at: http://www.pharmacoepi.org/policy/privacy.htm.

JHITA (Joint Healthcare Information Technology Alliance). Advocacy Paper: Medical Records Confidentiality Legislation [Web Page]. Available at: http://www.jhita.org/medical.htm.

Lo, Bernard, and Alpers, Ann. Uses and Abuses of Prescription Drug Information in Pharmacy Benefits Management Programs. JAMA. 2000 Feb 9; 283(6):801–806.

Lowrance, William W. Privacy and Health Research: A Report to the U.S. Secretary of Health and Human Services. 1997 May.

Nelson, Andrew F., Quiter, Elaine S., and Solberg, Leif I. The State of Research Within Managed Care Plans: 1997 Survey. Health Affairs. 1998 Jan–1998 Feb; 17(1):128–138.

NRC (National Research Council). Committee on Maintaining Privacy and Security in Health Care Applications of the National Infrastructure, Computer Science and Telecommunications Board, Commission on Physical Sciences, Mathematics and Applications, and National Research Council. For the Record. Protecting Electronic Health Information. Washington, DC: National Academy Press. 1997.

NRC (National Research Council) Panel of Confidentiality and Data Access, George T. Duncan, Thomas B. Jabine, and Virginia A. de Wolf, editors. Private Lives and Public Policies Confidentiality and Accessibility of Government Statistics. 1993.

O'Brien, Dale G., and Yasnoff, William A. Privacy, Confidentiality, and Security in Information Systems of State Health Agencies. American Journal of Preventive Medicine. 1999; 16(4):351–358.

OPRR, National Institute of Health. Intitutional Review Board (IRB) Guidebook, 1993 [Web Page]. 1993. Available at: http://grants.nih.gov/grants/oprr/irb/irb_guidebook.htm.

PhRMA. PhRMA Policy Papers: Twin Goals: Privacy and Progress [Web Page]. Available at: http://www.phrma.org/issues/goals.html.

Shalala, Donna. Confidentiality of Individually Identifiable Health Information, Recommendations of the Secretary of Health and Human Services, pursuant to section 264 of the Health Insurance Portability and Accountability Act of 1996. 1997 Sep 11.

Wiederhold, Gio. Traveling the Electronic Highway: Glossary Maps, Encounters, Directions. Terms relevant to Internet Computing. 1998 Jan.

Wolf, Leslie E. and Lo, Bernard. Practicing Safer Research Using the Law to Protect the Confidentiality of Sensitive Research Data.

ADDENDUM A

Workshop Speakers

Robert Amdur, M.D.
Associate Professor and Associate
   Chairman for Clinical Affairs
Department of Radiation Oncology
University of Florida Health Sciences
   Center

Arthur Anderson, M.D.
Fort Detrick, U.S. Army
Chief, Department of Clinical
   Pathology and Office of Human
   Use and Ethics
U.S. Army Medical Research
   Institute of Infectious Disease

Tora Bikson, Ph.D.
Senior Behavioral Scientist
Chair, IRB
RAND

Angela Bowen, M.D.
President
Western Institutional Review Board

Lawrence Dietz, Esq.
Market Intelligence Director
AXENT Technologies, Inc.

William Freeman, M.D., M.P.H.
Director, I.H.S. Research Program
Chair, Headquarters I.H.S. IRB
Rockville, MD

Steven A. Garfinkel, Ph.D.
Associate Director
Health Services and Policy Research
   Program
Research Triangle Institute

Harry Guess, Ph.D.
Chief, Epidemiology
Merck

Brent James, M.D.
Vice President for Medical Research
   and Continuing Medical Education
Intermountain Health Care

James Kahn, M.D.
Institute for Health Policy Studies
Department of Medicine,
University of California, San
    Francisco

S. Angela Khan
Institutional Coordinator, Research
    Review
Institutional Review Board
University of Texas Health Science
    Center at San Antonio

Bartha-Maria Knoppers, J.D.
Professor, Faculty of Law
Senior Researcher, C.R.D.P.
Legal Counsel, McMaster Gervais
University of Montreal

Morris Linton, JD
Senior Council
Intermountain Health Care

Jennifer Low, Esq.
Associate General Counsel
Express Scripts, Inc.

Andrew Nelson
Executive Director, HealthPartners
President, HMO Research Network
Minneapolis, MN

Thomas Puglisi, Ph.D.
Director, Division of Human Subjects
    Protections
Office for Protection from Research
    Risks
U.S. Department of Health and
    Human Services

Fred Teitelbaum, Ph.D
Vice President
Outcomes Research and Cost
    Management
Express Scripts, Health Management
    Services

Ross A. Thompson, Ph.D.
Professor
Department of Psychology
University of Nebraska

Workshop Participants

Olga Boikess
NIMH

Brian Brown
National Naval Medical Center
Institutional Review Board

Ruth Bulger
USUHS

Donna T. Chen
Southeastern Rural Mental Health
Research Center, University of
Virginia

Angela Choy
Institute for Health Care Research
and Policy
Georgetown University

Sarah Comley

Carrie Crawford
National Naval Medical Center
Institutional Review Board

Trenita Davis
National Institutes of Health (NIH)
National Institute of Dental and
Craniofacial Research

Nancy Donovan
U.S General Accounting Office
(GAO)

Gary B. Ellis
Office for Protection from Research
Risks
National Institutes of Health

John P. Fanning
Office of the Assistant Secretary for
Planning and Evaluation

Michael Fitzmaurice
Agency for Healthcare Research and
Quality

158

PROTECTING DATA PRIVACY

Ellen Gadbois
National Bioethics Advisory
    Commission

Olga Garcia
Office of Management and Budget

Felix Gyi
Chesapeake Research Review, Inc.

Stephen Heinig
Association of American Medical
    Colleges

Tom Hogan
The Blue Sheet

Julie Kaneshiro
National Institutes of Health

Richard A. Knazek
National Institutes of Health

Eric Larson
General Accounting Office

Richard Levine
USUHS

Joanne Lynn
RAND

Margaret Matula
National Institutes of Health

Laurie Michel
Merck

Mary Otto
Knight Ridder

Shannon Penberthy
Association for Health Services
    Research

Douglas Peddicord
Washington Health Advocates

Joan Porter
ORCA

Maryann Redford
National Institutes of Health

Patricia M. Scannell
Washington University School of
    Medicine

Gerald S. Schatz
National Institutes of Health

Amy Schwarzhoff
Chesapeake Research Review, Inc.

Ann Skinner
Johns Hopkins School of Public
    Health

Stuart F. Spicker
Massachusetts College of Pharmacy,
    Boston

Miron Straff
National Research Council

Bernard Talbat
National Institutes of Health

Ron Warren

Protecting the Health Services Research Data of Minors

Ross A. Thompson, Ph.D.

There are many issues relevant to the confidentiality, security, and privacy of personally identifiable health information (PHI) used for health services research purposes. These include (1) the nature of the confidentiality protections of privately funded health services research studies (which are not generally subject to institutional review board [IRB] approval), (2) the purposes for which the data were originally gathered, (3) the purposes for which they are used in secondary reanalysis, (4) the nature of the consent procedures originally used and the confidentiality assurances that are part of the consent process, (5) protections of the data while the study is under way, and (6) who the relevant actors and agencies fundamental to such procedures are (e.g., hospital IRBs, insurance companies managed care providers, physicians researchers).

These are difficult issues that are relevant to the PHI of all research participants, regardless of developmental stage. For example, problems of confidentiality emerge in very large databases when health events of extremely low frequency are studied and data relevant to these particular cases can easy lead to their identification. The steps that can be taken to ensure the confidentiality of health data such as these are unlikely to vary significantly depending on whether the health events beset adults or infants (e.g., a multiply challenged baby in the neonatal intensive care unit).

However, when children are research participants, there may be more unique risks to the confidentiality and privacy of their PHI and special concerns in the secondary analysis of their health data. This paper is devoted to framing the issues associated with protecting the health services research data of minors in light of how the PHI of minors is commonly treated in health services research. In brief summary, these include the following issues:

• Children constitute a heterogeneous population. Within the broad population of legally defined "minors," research studies document considerable variability in developing judgment, self-understanding, and psychosocial functioning. This means that:

    • the capacities of children and youth to assent to the uses of their PHI and to meaningfully understand assurances concerning confidentiality, privacy, and research risk develop considerably with increasing age, with adultlike capabilities evident early in adolescence;
    • the psychological risks posed by the inappropriate disclosure of minors' PHI (e.g., perceived privacy violations, feelings of embarrassment or humiliation, threats to their medical or legal interests) change complexly with development but, by late childhood, approximate the risks experienced by adults;
    • in longitudinal studies, and in the secondary analysis of previously collected PHI, older children and adolescents may be concerned about access to health data collected when they were younger and have a strong interest in giving independent consent to its use.

These considerations are relevant to all minors, especially to adolescent populations who can in some jurisdictions consent independently of their parents to certain forms of medical treatment (e.g., substance abuse or mental health treatment).

• Children constitute a uniquely vulnerable population because of their limited rights under the law and their limited capacities for autonomous decision making. This means that special provisions are needed to ensure their protection from research risks, which include, but extend beyond, parental proxy consent on their behalf.

• Problems in proxy consent arise from (1) fundamental difficulties in distinguishing the interests of children from those of their parents or other custodians, (2) the fact that consent also involves accepting provisions for control over research materials, knowledge of research findings, and conditions governing children's elective withdrawal from research participation in which parents' and children's interests may also differ, and (3) lack of clarity about whether proxy consent endures for the entire course of the research investigation, including longitudinal or secondary analyses, regardless of children's developing capacities (and interests) in asserting and protecting their own rights as research participants as they mature.

• Special considerations in biomedical data result from the uniquely sensitive nature of such data, and the potential immediate and longer-term implications of PHI for children in the context of family dynamics. These require immediate determinations about who has access to, and control over, children's PHI that take into consideration life-course concerns for children.

Taken together, it is clear that the health information of minors should be considered very differently from the PHI of adults in a manner that reflects their developing capabilities and a life-span consideration of children's interests.

A CASE ILLUSTRATION

These issues related to protection of the research data of minors are not exclusive to PHI. To illustrate, consider the following hypothetical case study (based on actual published research):

A research team inaugurates a large, longitudinal study of children's social and emotional adjustment in the 1970s. This research enlists a representative sample of more than 2,000 children in the early gradeschool years from a large urban population. Passive consent procedures are used (i.e., parents receive a letter describing the nature of the study and are asked to contact the investigators if they wish their child NOT to participate). The children are assessed annually on six occasions after the study begins, with assessments including measures of peer relationships, self-perceptions, academic competence, and emotional functioning.

Fifteen years after the study begins, a new researcher joins the team with interests in the prediction of child maltreatment. After obtaining IRB approval, the names and other identifying information of children in the original research are matched against the state's child abuse registry, after permission to do so is obtained from state officials. This results in a large sample of children identified as having been abused or neglected when the original research was in progress. Furthermore, the social service agencies for counties in the area are contacted and invited to participate in the research by sharing the child protective services case records of the identified children in the sample. Based on these records, the timing, type, chronicity, and severity of maltreatment is determined. Careful efforts are taken to ensure the confidentiality of all research materials.

As a consequence, a uniquely informative investigation of the antecedents and correlates of child maltreatment using a prospective longitudinal design with a large, representative sample results. Matched subsamples of maltreated and nonmaltreated children are compared to address fundamental questions about the impact of the experience of abuse or neglect, and its timing and severity, on various measures of psychosocial and emotional adjustment in childhood.

A number of questions are raised by this case illustration that are also relevant to the protection of health services research data by minors:

- Given the sensitive nature of the secondary analyses (and potential perceptions of privacy invasion), were the researchers ethically obligated to seek permission from families in the study when the investigation later turned to the prediction of child maltreatment? Or did the original consent procedures apply to the secondary data analysis that also involved accessing confidential state records?

• Did the initial use of parental passive consent procedures—rather than active consent, in which the parent must contact the researchers to consent volitionally after having been informed about the research purposes—alter the ethical obligation to seek further consent after the research team began to investigate more sensitive issues? Or were original consent procedures adequate regardless of whether passive or active consent was used?

• Because a significant proportion of the children originally enlisted into the study had reached the age of majority before the secondary analyses began, were the researchers ethically obligated to contact them for permission to use data gathered during their minority? Or were the original consent procedures, involving parents but not children, still sufficient at this later period?

• Without opportunities for further informed consent, was it possible for the participant families or children (now, in some cases, young adults), to protect themselves against the potential risks involved in the secondary analyses of these data in concert with protected (and confidential) state records?

ISSUES TO CONSIDER

There are no easy answers to these questions, but posing them thoughtfully is essential to consider judgments about how the needs and rights of minors can be protected in health services research data that may be subjected to secondary analysis. There are additional considerations, discussed below, that add further complexity to thinking about any potential special ethical review requirements of research involving minors.

Children as a Heterogeneous Population

Although the term "children" is commonly used in these contexts to refer to all persons below the age of majority, it is instructive to realize that the term encompasses infants, preschoolers, gradeschool children, and adolescents within a single conceptual umbrella. Although the umbrella may be sufficient for legal purposes, it ill-fits the heterogeneity of capabilities, interests, and needs characterizing the population it covers.

With respect to the reflective judgment required for informed consent, for example, there is considerable research evidence that by early adolescence, young people are capable of making informed consent decisions about medical treatment and research participation that are comparable in quality to those of adults (Abramovitch et al., 1995; Abramovitch et al., 1991; Lewis et al., 1978; Melton et al., 1983; Ruck et al., 1998; Ruck et al., 1998; Weithorn, 1982, 1983; Weithorn and Campbell, 1982). At somewhat earlier ages (i.e., during the gradeschool years), children's informed consent capabilities are more uneven or inconsistent, although their judgment can be strengthened through the use of simple interventions, such as providing short, educational information about rights and prerogatives as a research participant (Abramovitch et al., 1995; Rau and Fisher, 1999). Thus, the capacities of children to assert an active, responsible voice in judgments concerning their research participation increases significantly with age, with mature competence reached well before the legal age of majority, but with the capacity for mature consent strengthened through age-appropriate educational interventions.

In a somewhat comparable manner, the psychological risks to which children are vulnerable also change significantly with age. Moreover, these risks change in complex ways: some decrease with increasing age, others increase as children mature, and still others remain essentially stable over the course of development (Thompson, 1990a, b, 1992). This challenges the prevailing assumption that children become less vulnerable in research contexts as they mature. For example, although children become progressively less prone with increasing age to becoming distressed, overwhelmed, or disorganized in research settings because of the development of emotional and behavioral self-regulation and coping skills, children become *more* susceptible to other risks from their research participation as they mature. These include susceptibility to threats to self-concept and self-esteem (sometimes arising from performance evaluation),; vulnerability to feelings of shame, embarrassment, or humiliation (sometimes from concerns about the improper disclosure of personal information); and concern about expressed or implied social comparison evaluations. Likewise, although children become progressively less prone to being deceived or coerced by research procedures as they develop more mature and insightful judgment about the motives of other people, they also become more vulnerable to concern about perceived privacy violations in the use of their research data. Indeed, for many adolescents, concerns with personal privacy extend to the disclosure of personal information, such as their research data, even to parents (see Wolfe, 1978).

There are several implications of this developmental analysis of research risk:

- The psychological risks associated with research participation and deriving from the imroper disclosure of research data vary as minors mature, but do not necessarily decrease linearly with increasing age. For some risks, vulnerability increases. Moreover, children's vulnerability to the research risks most pertinent to adults increases sharply over time; these include perceived violations of privacy, the embarrassment and humiliation that may derive from inappropriate disclosure of personal health data, and some of the tangible consequences of unwarranted disclosure (e.g., difficult family processes or compromised medical or legal circumstances; see below).

- Estimating the nature of the research risks to which children are vulnerable is thus a developmentally graded assessment, and in longitudinal research these risks may change as children mature over the course of the investigation. In other words, the research risks relevant to an investigation that was inaugurated when children were preschoolers are not necessarily the same as those relevant by the time the same children have become adolescents. This means that a revised risk–benefit calculus becomes necessary as longitudinal research proceeds (Thompson, 1992).

• In the secondary analysis of data (as with longitudinal data), the constellation of risks to which children are vulnerable is also likely to change with the passage of time since the original data were gathered. In addition, older children and adolescents, like young adults, are likely to feel much differently about the uses of data gathered when they were very young than they were capable of feeling at the time these data were initially obtained. Concerns over personal privacy, threats of embarrassment or humiliation, and more tangible concerns related to the potentially inappropriate disclosure of research data now become personal issues (whereas formerly they were addressed on behalf of the child through parental proxy consent procedures).

Any assessment of the ethical responsibilities of researchers should take these developmentally changing concerns into consideration.

Children as a Uniquely Vulnerable Population

A longstanding tradition of special protections for children and youth in research derives from the special configuration of child, parental, and state interests related to children's research participation. Within moral theory, the unique characteristics of children account for their limited self-determination and the beneficent paternalism they receive from others (Baumrind, 1978; Melton, 1987). Their limited experience and immature reasoning capabilities together mean that although children (as persons before the law) are entitled to some of the rights of privacy and self-determination granted to adults, their capacities to exercise these rights are limited. They are limited, in part, because of the responsibilities entrusted to others to safeguard their welfare. As a consequence, adults (especially parents) make fundamental decisions concerning the research participation of their offspring, exercising proxy consent on behalf of children and making other decisions concerning research on behalf of their children's interests. Moreover, the state also assumes a special interest in the child's well-being, independently of the authority of parents, because of its responsibility under the *parens patriae* doctrine. This is one reason why the ethical review of research protocols involving children by state-appointed agencies (e.g., IRBs) is typically more searching, even though parents also exercise proxy consent on behalf of their offspring.

This means that children are almost uniquely powerless social actors in decisions concerning their research participation and the disposition of their research materials. Although children's assent is encouraged by existing federal regulations, it may be difficult for them to dissent meaningfully from research participation not only because of limitations in judgment, but also because their invitation to participate typically occurs in a context of prior parental permission, institutional support (whether the institution is a school, childcare center, hospital, or other setting), and adults' interests in furthering the research enterprise (Abramovitch et al., 1991). For the same reasons, children's social power to resist research procedures that they find unduly distressing, psychologically invasive, or coercive may also be quite limited. Furthermore, children experience limited social power not only over decisions concerning their research participation but also over other elements of the research process, such as the disclosure of research data and assurances concerning the disposition of research materials, their withdrawal from research participation after the study has begun, and obtaining the benefits (if any) of research participation. Each of these ordinary prerogatives of the research participant is exercised instead by adults as proxies for the child.

Of course, in most cases, adults (especially parents) make decisions in the interests of children. However, it is unwise to assume that the interests of parents and offspring are always identical in these situations and that the motives underlying parental consent are always consistent with children's interests. Recognizing this, the federal regulations governing research with children (Department of Health and Human Services [DHHS], 1991) not only require special review considerations in studies involving children, but also encourage the child's assent to research participation when children are capable of doing so meaningfully. (Indeed, in 1978 the National Commission for the Protection of Human Subjects of Biomedical and Behavioral Research recommended that a child's objection to research participation constitute a *binding* restriction except in extraordinary circumstances and that the assent of children age 7 and older be required for their research participation. These provisions were not, however, incorporated into the final DHHS regulations.) These provisions seem to reflect the following: (1) children's unique needs and social vulnerability mandate special consideration in the ethical review of research, (2) adults (usually parents) must exercise proxy consent on behalf of children, but (3) proxy consent alone cannot be the only assurance that children are not subject to unreasonable risk. These provisions raise further the question of whether, when data gathered on an earlier occasion are enlisted later into new research purposes (e.g., secondary or longitudinal analyses), children should be capable of making their own, independent decisions concerning access to and the disposition of their research materials if they have developed sufficiently mature judgment to do so.

Problems in Proxy Consent

Just as there is value in recognizing that parents usually make thoughtful judgments concerning the research participation of their offspring, there is value also in recognizing the circumstances in which proxy consent does not necessarily protect children's interests. When parents derive financial benefit, access to services, or other personal rewards from the research participation of offspring for example, proxy consent may not adequately protect children's interests. (Indeed, philosopher Paul Ramsay, 1970, 1976, 1977 has argued that *any* nontherapeutic research with children is morally impermissible because even proxy consent inevitably confounds adults' interests with those of children.) In abusive or adversarial parent–child relationships, adults may be motivated to deny permission if children's research participation might contribute to the detection of maltreatment, substance abuse, or other parental problems. With respect to medical research (e.g., PHI), proxy consent by parents may be problematic in situations when biological assessments of offspring are needed to evaluate the medical condition of another family member (e.g., in genetic screening studies or DNA analysis of tissue samples), or parents may be motivated to conduct risk assessment (presymptomatic) testing of offspring for disorders that are not immediately relevant to the child's well-being (e.g., Huntington's disease).

Potential problems in proxy consent are even more apparent when consent is given not by a biological parent, but by a representative of a government agency when children are wards of the state (see National Bioethics Advisory Commission, 1998). In these circumstances, inappropriate incentives may result in considerable pressure for children to participate in research studies that may not be in their best interests.

In some situations, adolescents may be hesitant to obtain parental consent for medical treatment of sensitive conditions (e.g., substance abuse or mental health problems) because of privacy concerns. Current legal policies in many states recognize this in allowing adolescents to consent independently to certain forms of treatment without parental consent. This raises important issues concerning the confidentiality of medical records arising from treatment and adolescents' control over the disclosure of this information to family members and others outside the family. Likewise, behavioral researchers have long recognized that parental consent may be an impediment to research participation by older children and adolescents in research studies of sensitive topics (e.g., sexuality, drug or alcohol use) in which parental consent is also likely to violate the privacy interests of youth. In these circumstances, confidentiality and the control over access to research data must also be carefully considered.

The potential problems of proxy consent are magnified somewhat by two additional considerations. First, consent also typically includes accepting provisions for and assurance of responsibility for many other aspects of research participation in which parents and children's interests may not be identical. These include, for example, provisions governing access to the research data gathered from children, issues of privacy and confidentiality of research materials, children's knowledge of the results of the research inquiry, and conditions governing children's elective withdrawal from research participation. In certain situations, the decisions of parents may be influenced by factors different from those relevant to children's needs and interests.

Second, consent is often assumed to endure for the duration of the research investigation. As noted earlier, this may be problematic in longitudinal studies or in the secondary analysis of original data that occurs at which children have matured to an age when their own independent judgments concerning the disposition of their research data are relevant. Children's independent consent is important not only to respect their increasing maturity concerning judgments about research participation (and their rights as research participants), but to enable them independently to protect their prerogatives as research participants by participating in a consent process in which provisions about confidentiality and privacy, risks and benefits, freedom to withdraw and access to research findings are discussed.

In light of these considerations, it becomes apparent also why many research scientists believe that passive consent procedures are inappropriate to research involving children (e.g., Fisher, 1993). In passive consent, parents receive notice of a research study in which their children will participate unless the parent contacts the investigator to prohibit participation. By contrast, active consent procedures require the parent's volitional consent before children can participate in research. The fundamental problem with passive consent procedures is the assumption that parents who do not respond have assented to research participation when, in fact, they may have failed to receive relevant information, it may have been lost or misplaced after it was received, or parents may have otherwise neglected to indicate their objections to their child's research involvement. Passive consent is also problematic because entailed in the consent process is the acceptance of many other provisions governing research participation (e.g., provisions concerning disclosure, confidentiality, and protection of research data; conditions governing children's withdrawal from research participation; assurances concerning risks and benefits from research involvement; and guarantees concerning penalties owing to the failure to participate in research) for which active, not passive, consent is necessary. Active consent is especially important in situations where parents are acting as proxies in protecting their children's needs and interests.

For similar reasons, blanket research consent provisions incorporated into insurance and consent-to-treatment documents that permit PHI (and, quite often, the PHI of family members) to be used for secondary research purposes may be equally inappropriate from the perspective of research ethics. Without clear information concerning the nature of the secondary research purposes and relevant assurances concerning privacy and confidentiality, it is difficult for an individual to know what he or she is consenting to. Moreover, when such blanket consent is requested at the time of medical treatment, these circumstances may make it very difficult to decline.

Special Considerations in Biomedical Data

The need for parental proxy consent and children's assent, the developmentally graded risks faced by children owing to the inappropriate disclosure of research data, and the growing capacities for personally informed consent that emerge as minors mature are considerations shared by behavioral and biomedical researchers who enlist children into their studies. There are, however, a number of concerns that are more specific to health services research data, such as those used for secondary research purposes, because of the broader implications of the data for children and their families (see, generally, National Bioethics Advisory Commission, 1999). These make considerations associated with the control and dissemination of PHI especially germane, particularly when data are collected and/or used by agencies not usually governed by the Common Rule. These issues can be illustrated by considering the genetic testing of children and adolescents.

With the recent significant advances in knowledge generated by the Human Genome Project, the challenges posed by the uses and potential misuses of personal genetic information have received increased attention. Genetic testing of children and youth can occur for many reasons, as in genetic screening or pedigree analyses (e.g., to trace the family history of a disease) or in DNA analysis of tissue samples for research or therapeutic purposes. As knowledge of the human genome increases, it is likely that genetic testing of children will increase in the years to come. Whatever the reasons that testing initially occurs, genetic testing may yield information of a sensitive nature for children and adolescents, such as the discovery of an inherited vulnerability, possibly for a stigmatizing (e.g., mental illness, alcoholism) or life-threatening disease (e.g., Huntington's disease, cancer).

There are immediate and long-term implications of the knowledge yielded by genetic testing of children and adolescents that are directly relevant to the dissemination and confidentiality of the results of their testing. In the immediate context, knowledge of inherited vulnerabilities can be distressing and confusing, especially given the uncertain, probabilistic prognostic implications of this information (indeed, most adults are unlikely to grasp the indeterminate implications of a genetic marker for an inherited disorder). This requires sensitive considerations of whether children and youth are permitted access to their testing results, conditions under which this information is provided, and the availability of support and guidance to help ensure that youth respond constructively (e.g., by enlisting pathology-preventive behavioral practices, if possible) rather than nonconstructively (e.g., through personally abusive practices or the development of depressive or anxious pathology) to the news that they have an inherited vulnerability (Gardner et al., 1992). This might involve enlisting a fellow health care professional, a trusted extended family member, or an adult friend, to discuss distressing health care findings with an adolescent when immediate family members may not be the most suitable counselors, perhaps because of their own conflicts or interest or owing to family dissension.

These considerations lead to a series of important questions. Who else is allowed access to the information yielded by a child's or an adolescent's genetic testing? Who decides if, when, and how the young person is provided with this knowledge? To what extent are the youth's preferences to know—or not know—the results of the test determinative at the time the testing is conducted or in the future? To what extent does a child or adolescent have control over whether this information is shared with family members or with others outside the family? There is value in creative avenues for protecting children while also ensuring that their privacy and self-determination are safeguarded. One research

team, for example, protected adolescents' "right not to know" the results of genetic test for Huntington's disease, but also put the testing results in a registry to
which youth would have direct and exclusive access after age 18 (see Fisher et
al., 1996).

These questions are important because of their relevance to the potential
extended implications of the information yielded by genetic testing. In a long-
term context, knowledge of inherited vulnerabilities can have implications for
employment, insurability, and health care coverage that may be based on an
accurate or inaccurate understanding of the broader implications of markers
within the genotype for inherited disorders. This raises similar questions about
the control of the information yielded by a young person's genetic testing and
the importance of guarding against the risks inherent in the unwarranted (and
unwanted) disclosure of personal health information such as this, especially for
institutions not typically governed by the Common Rule. Importantly, PHI improperly disseminated during a child's minority can have longer-term implications for that person's well-being after he or she has become an adult.

The secondary analysis of health care data adds further questions to these.
This arises, in part, because as children mature to majority age, they may be
entitled to an active role in decisions concerning the use of their original testing
results. Furthermore, the interests that governed initial parental proxy consent to
genetic testing may be much different from those governing the young adult's
personal concerns about the dissemination of this information. This suggests that
procedures governing the uses of PHI obtained from minors must be considered
within a life-span context for the individual. The consent processes and assurances that occurred at the time a child was initially tested may not generalize to
later conditions in which the adolescent or young adult can better represent her
or his own interests and preferences, and may have an interest in doing so.

CONCLUSIONS

A central challenge in considering the ethics of research with children is the
juxtaposition of the interests of children, their parents, and the research community within the context of children's limited decision-making capabilities and
our cultural commitment to beneficent paternalism on their behalf (e.g., Koocher
and Keith-Spiegel, 1990). When considering how best to protect the health
services research data of minors, especially in the context of the secondary
analysis of these data, the issues become especially complex because of the
changing developmental needs and interests of minors over the course of the
investigation, which may be very different at the time of the secondary analysis
of data than they were at the time the data were originally gathered (and consent
procedures were originally instituted). These problems are encountered, in
somewhat different ways, by behavioral researchers who conduct longitudinal
studies in which children's involvement in research is maintained through their
increasingly active participation in decision-making on their behalf as they mature. In biomedical research most relevant to PHI, however, the challenges are

additionally complicated because family needs can be confounded with children's needs, the dissemination of children's PHI can create family conflict, health care institutions may or may not be governed by traditional procedures associated with protection from research risks, and the inappropriate disclosure of children's PHI can have lifelong implications for children that affect them well after they have reached the age of majority.

With respect to the practices of IRBs in their review of research protocols involving children, several kinds of questions are warranted.

- Do research procedures undergo a more searching examination when children are research participants, particularly with respect to assessing in a developmentally graded manner the potential risks of their research participation? IRBs assume a special responsibility to children as research participants and cannot assume that parental proxy consent will always safeguard children's interests.

- Are active parental consent procedures used when children are below the age of majority? Are consent procedures sufficiently specific and clear that parents can make reasonable judgments concerning the nature of the research procedures and the uses of research data?

- Do research procedures provide for children's assent to research participation independent of parental consent? Are these procedures appropriate to the child's age and conducted in a manner that avoids undue incentives or pressure on the child? Do these procedures attempt to provide information to children, suitable to their understanding of their rights concerning the privacy and confidentiality of the information yielded by research, their freedom to withdraw from participation, and related prerogatives? (Some IRBs require documentation of the proportion of children who do not assent to research procedures and who seek to withdraw from participation once the research has begun.)

- With older children and adolescents, do research procedures provide for their active participation in the process of research consent, recognizing the maturity of their independent judgment?

- When research is longitudinal in nature or when secondary analyses of previously collected data are conducted, is a follow-up IRB review needed to determine whether additional consent procedures are required from the children who participated in the original research or from their parents? Are there new dimensions of potential research risk arising from the fact that the children are now older or from changes in research purposes or goals?

- When sensitive data (e.g., the results of biomedical assessments) are obtained, is thoughtful consideration devoted to questions such as (1) who has access to this information, (2) whether, and under what circumstances, the child or adolescent is informed about testing results; and (3) provisions for the child to obtain direct access to this information, and control over its dissemination, after reaching the age of majority?

As a general rule, it is valuable to consider the protection of health services research data for minors within a life-span context, taking into consideration the longer-term implications of decisions made early on behalf of the child, as well as the child's own preferences and goals (Fisher, 1997). Procedures that respect children's immediate and long-term interests in the privacy, confidentiality, and protection of their PHI, in the context of respecting their rights to age-appropriate self-determination, are especially warranted.

REFERENCES

Abramovitch, R., Freedman, J. L., Henry, K., and Van Brunschot, M. (1995). Children's capacity to agree to psychological research: Knowledge of risks and benefits and voluntaries. *Ethics and Behavior, 5*, 25–48.

Abramovitch, R., Freedman, J. L., Thoden, K., and Nikolich, C. (1991). Children's capacity to consent to participation in psychological research: Empirical findings. *Child Development, 62,* 1100–1109.

Baumrind, D. (1978). Reciprocal rights and responsibilities in parent–child relations. *Journal of Social Issues, 34,* 179–196.

Department of Health and Human Services (DHHS) (1991). *Code of Federal Regulations. Protection of Human Subjects.* 45 CFR 46, Subparts A and D. Washington, DC: U.S.Government Printing Office.

Fisher, C. B. (1993). Integrating science and ethics in research with high risk children and youth. *Social Policy Report of the Society for Research in Child Development, 7,* 1–27.

Fisher, C. B. (1997). A relational perspective on ethics-in-science decisionmaking for research with vulnerable populations. *IRB: A Review of Human Subjects Research, 19,* 1–4.

Fisher, C. B., Hoagwood, K., and Jensen, P. S. (1996). Casebook on ethical issues in research with children and adolescents with mental disorders. In K. Hoagwood, P. S. Jensen, and C. B. Fisher (Eds.), *Ethical Issues in Mental Health Research with Children and Adolescents.* Pp. 135–266. Mahwah, NJ: Erlbaum.

Gardner, W., Thompson, R. A., and Smith, M. G. (1992, April). *Genetic Counseling About Risks of Chronic Diseases: Developmental Perspectives on Adolescents' Best Interests and Legal Rights.* In E. J. Susman (chair), *Ethical Issues and the adolescent: Research, Health Care, and Social Policy.* Symposium conducted at the meeting of the Society for Research on Adolescence, New Orleans, LA.

Koocher, G. P., and Keith-Spiegel, P. C. (1990). *Children, Ethics, and the Law.* Lincoln, NE: University of Nebraska Press.

Lewis, C. E., Lewis, M. A., and Ifekwunigue, M. (1978). Informed consent by children and participation in an influenza vaccine trial. *American Journal of Public Health, 68,* 1079–1082.

Melton, G. B. (1987). The clashing of symbols: Prelude to child and family policy. *American Psychologist, 42,* 345–354.

Melton, G. B., Koocher, G. P., and Saks, M. J. (Eds.) (1983). *Children's Competence to Consent.* New York: Plenum.

National Bioethics Advisory Commission (1998). *Research Involving Persons with Mental Disorders That May Affect Decisionmaking Capacity.* Rockville, MD.

National Bioethics Advisory Commission (1999). *Research Involving Human Biological Materials: Ethical Issues and Policy Guidance.* Vol. 1. *Report and Recommendations of the National Bioethics Advisory Commission.* Rockville, MD.

Ramsay, P. (1970). *The Patient as Person.* New Haven: Yale University Press.

Ramsay, P. (1976). The enforcement of morals: Nontherapeutic research on children. *Hastings Center Report,* August, 21–30.

Ramsay, P. (1977). Children as research subjects: A reply. *Hastings Center Report,* April, 40–42.

Rau, J.-M. B., and Fisher, C. B. (1999). *Assessing and Enhancing the Research Consent Capacity of Children and Youth.* Unpublished manuscript, Department of Psychology, Fordham University, New York.

Ruck, M. D., Abramovitch, R., and Keating, D.P. (1998 a). Children's and adolescents' understanding of rights: Balancing nurturance and self-determination. *Child Development, 64,* 404–417.

Ruck, M. D., Keating, D. P., Abramovitch, R., and Koegl, C. J. (1998 b). Adolescents' and children's knowledge about rights: Some evidence for how young people view rights in their own lives. *Journal of Adolescence, 21,* 275–289.

Thompson, R. A. (1990a). Vulnerability in research: A developmental perspective on research risk. *Child Development, 61,* 1–16.

Thompson, R. A. (1990b). Behavioral research involving children: A developmental perspective on risk. *IRB: A Review of Human Subjects Research, 12,* 1–6.

Thompson, R. A. (1992). Developmental changes in research risk and benefit: A changing calculus of concerns. B. Stanley and J. E. Sieber (Eds.), *Social Research on Children and Adolescents: Ethical Issues.* (Pp. 31–64). Newbury Park, CA: Sage.

Weithorn, L. A. (1982). Developmental factors and competence to make informed treatment decisions. Pp. 85–100 G. B. Melton , *Legal Reforms Affecting Child and Youth Services* New York: Haworth.

Weithorn, L. A. (1983). Children's capacities to decide about participation in research. *IRB: A Review of Human Subjects Research, 5,* 1–5.

Weithorn, L. A., and Campbell, S. B. (1982). The competency of children and adolescents to make informed consent treatment decisions. *Child Development, 53,* 1589–1598.

Wolfe, M. (1978). Childhood and privacy. Pp. 175–222 I. Altman and J. F. Wohlwill (Eds.), Children and the Environment. New York: Plenum.

Confidentiality of Health Information: International Comparative Approaches

Bartha Maria Knoppers, J.D.

Although the concept of the confidentiality of personal medical data is well accepted by the general public and by health professionals, the detailed practice is under potentially serious attack by governments that want access in order to combat fraud or serious crime or to improve efficiency of services, by big business that wishes to improve its competitive edge or reduce its costs by utilizing detailed personal data in order to focus the promotion of its products and services, and by health care organizations that do not keep their security measures up to the state of the art required by the information processing facilities available and the attacks on personal medical data.[1]

A brief comparative overview of international and national developments on the confidentiality of health information over the last half century must of needs cover (1) the right of privacy, (2) medical confidentiality *per se,* and (3) the protection of personal data. Together they overlap and sometimes commingle. Whether understood as a property or liberty interest,[2] privacy continues to develop the zone of personal intimacy free from public scrutiny. Medical confidentiality arises from both the nature of the information concerned and the fiduciary character of the physician/ patient relationship. It has seen a movement towards greater patient as opposed to professional control of health information. Finally, the recent appearance of personal data protection laws not only shields the individual from the powers of informatics but also provides a measure of security and personal control. Privacy, confidentiality, and personal data protection are inseparable when touching upon health information.

INTERNATIONAL

In 1948, the United Nations adopted article 12 of the *Universal Declaration,* which upholds the protection against "arbitrary interference with [one's] privacy, family, home or correspondence" and "attacks upon [one's] honor and

---

[1]Barber, B., "Patient Data and Security: An Overview" (1998) 49 *International Journal of Medical Informatics,* 19 at 25.

[2]Le Bris, S., and B.M. Knoppers, "International and Comparative Concepts of Privacy" in Rothstein, M. (ed.) *Genetic Secrets* New Haven: Yale University Press, (1997) 418–448.

reputation." This same right is also found in the 1955 European Convention on Human Rights, although the possibility of State "interference"... "for the protection of health" was specifically foreseen as a possible exception. Although the right to privacy was further strengthened by its inclusion in the 1976 United Nations International Covenant on Civil and Political Rights, it was both the Council of Europe's 1981 Convention for the Protection of Individuals with Regard to the Automatic Processing of Data which considered health data as "special", and the Organization for Economic Cooperation and Development (OECD's) 1989 *Guidelines for the Protection of Privacy and Transborder Flows* that established the modern parameters for the principled regulation and security of medical data. The eight OECD principles are: (1) collection limitation; (2) data quality; (3) purpose specification; (4) use limitation; (5) security safeguards; (6) openness; (7) individual participation; and (8) accountability. The 1981 Convention, in particular, established exceptions for data banks for statistics or scientific research purposes as well as the rules for record linkage.

The last decade has also witnessed an increasing emphasis on patient autonomy and patient's rights. Thus, according to the World Health Organization, all health status information should remain confidential even after death (art. 4.1), *Declaration on the Promotion of Patient's Rights in Europe*). Concurrent with this expanding ambit of confidentiality is that of the notion of identifiability through personal data. The 1995 European Community *Directive on the Protection of Individuals* (with regard to the processing of personal data and on the free movement of such data) defines personal data as "any information relating to an individual or identifiable natural person "(data subject); an identifiable person is one who can be "identified, directly or indirectly, in particular by reference to an identification number or to one or more factors specific to his physical, physiological, mental, economic, cultural or social identity." (art. 2.a).

It was however, the 1997 Council of Europe's Convention on Human Rights and Biomedicine that included a new corollary right: "the right not to be informed about health information" within the concept of respect for private life and the right to information. In a sense, privacy in the health sector once associated with the property of medical records, then as a right of "secrecy" (i.e., not to be personally identified or "processed" without consent), has now been extended to cover the sphere of personal intimacy through not being informed of one's own health data.

In that same year, the Council of Europe also adopted Recommendation R97 (5) on the Protection of Medical Data. Three articles bear mention here:

Article 1. An individual shall not be regarded as 'identifiable' if identification requires an unreasonable amount of time and manpower.

Article 3.1. The respect of rights and fundamental freedoms, and in particular of the right to privacy, shall be guaranteed during the collection and processing of medical data.

Article 7.2. In particular, unless other appropriate safeguards are provided by domestic law, medical data may only be communicated to a person who is subject to the rules of confidentiality incumbent upon a health care professional, or to comparable rules of confidentiality, and who complies with the provisions of this recommendation.

The status of a Council of Europe's convention is that of an international treaty, and it is binding on signatory states. The first article cited above again takes up the challenge of defining identifiability in a computerized society, thus adding the proviso "requiring an unreasonable amount of time and manpower." The second makes explicit the link between privacy and medical data (which according to another article includes genetic data). The third limits the persons who can receive such data to health professionals or those "with comparable rules of confidentiality." This latter requirement resonates with the "extraterritoriality" approach of the 1995 European Community Directive mentioned earlier, which is binding on countries within the European Union (EU).

According to the Directive, not only must all 15 member States establish legislation that conforms with its standards, but personal data cannot be transferred from an EU country to a non-EU recipient country unless the protections in the recipient country are deemed to afford "adequate levels of protection" (art. 25.1).

The processing of health data is not distinguished from that of other personal data but the exemptions provided for under article 8 are certainly relevant:

Where processing of the data is required for the purposes of preventive medicine, medical diagnosis, the provision of care or treatment or the management of health care services, and where those data are processed by a health professional subject under national law or rules established by national competent bodies subject to the obligation of professional secrecy or by another person also subject to an equivalent obligation of secrecy.

Finally in 1999, the European Group on Ethics in Science and New Technologies issued an opinion *"Ethical Issues of Health Care in the Information Society."*[3] Not only are the eight principles broader than the OECD data principles, but participation and education have been added to the traditional list.

The group calls for a clear statement on rights and duties related to personal health data in the information society at a European level. Indeed, the opinion asserts that

1. A directive on medical data protection is desirable within the framework of the current Data Protection Directive to address particular issues arising from the use of health data;
2. A European patient's charter covering the above aspects, possibly by means of a recommendation, should be adopted.

---

[3]The principles are (1) privacy, (20) Confidentiality, (3) Principle of "legitimate purpose,"(4) consent, (5) security, (6) transparency, (7) participation, and (8) education.

In short, there are four well-established core information principles concerning personal data protection in Europe: 1) statutory protection; 2) transparent processing; 3) special protection for sensitive data, and, 4) enforcement rights for individuals. Nevertheless, a recent study for the OECD on "Data Protection in Trans-Border Flows of Health Research Data," while supportive of self-regulatory codes of conduct (especially where there is scrutiny by a data protection authority and eligibility for funding), emphasizes the need for more consolidation.[4] Within the area of sensitive data, health information is increasingly being singled out as being in need of specific statutory protection in spite of the application of the four core principles through a web of legal instruments. Nowhere is this trend more evident however than in national legislation.

NATIONAL

United Kingdom

In the United Kingdom (UK), confidentiality is afforded both Common Law and statutory protection. Beginning with the Common Law, "[i]t is generally thought that the action of breach of confidence is now a *sui generis* action finding its roots in principle of equity, contract, property and tort" Kennedy and Grubb, 1998; (p. 497),). The obligation of confidence arises both from the context in which the information is communicated to the doctor and from the nature of that relationship. Furthermore, "important public interests favor confidentiality where personal information is communicated in circumstances in which it is clear that the recipient is expected to respect the privacy of that information" (p. 502). In order to succeed in an action for breach of confidentiality, a plaintiff would have to show some form of injury (including mental distress) or economic loss (p. 514). Finally, contrary to Civil Law, a physician may disclose confidential information in the courtroom due to the public interest in the administration of justice, with the possibility that refusal could be considered contempt of court.

Common Law may be modified by statute. For example, the Data Protection Act of 1998 includes in its core principles the duty to process fairly and lawfully personal data. Sensitive data, defined as including health data, cannot be processed in the absence of explicit consent unless they are necessary for medical purposes or "undertaken by a professional who in the circumstances owes a duty of confidentiality which is equivalent to that which would arise if that person were a health professional" (Schedule 3, sec. 8).

It should be noted that the Human Rights Act (1998) incorporates the European Convention on Human Rights into UK law. This guarantees the right to

---

[4]Organization for Economic Cooperation and Development, *Data Protection in Transborder Flows of Health Research Data* (STI: Health Policy Brief) 1999, at p.23; See also Schwartz, P. "European Data Protection Law and Medical Privacy" in Rothstein, M. (ed.), *supra*, note 2, 392–417.

respect for privacy and family life. Superimposed on this, the previously mentioned Data Protection Act of 1998 provides a framework of rights and principles governing the use of electronic or structured paper records, including fair processing. Nevertheless, in spite of the core principles found therein, the law does not specify when confidential information should and should not be disclosed to others, in research or most other activities. Thus, decisions must be made according to Common Law on a case-by-case basis even when a research project has been approved by a Research ethics committee and authorized by a health authority.[5]

It also bears noting that in 1999, the British Medical Association (BMA) reiterated its request for statutory intervention to clarify the law in respect of the confidentiality of medical information in both the private and the state sector.[6]

The general principles put forward by the BMA follow:

- Information disclosed should be the minimum necessary to achieve the objective and, whenever possible, anonymous.
- Patients should be made aware of the potential uses of their information and be given an opportunity to object. Use of information for research is currently accepted as long as it is carried out within the guidelines and subject to monitoring by appropriately constituted research ethics committees. The BMA strongly recommends that patients be made aware that research is carried out and that it may involve the use of their records unless they object.

Generally, the association maintains that although research constitutes a justifiable use of personal health information, ideally it should use anonymized data wherever possible. The information disclosed should be the minimum necessary to achieve the objective. It may be possible to use pseudonyms or other tracking mechanisms for information, which cannot be anonymized, thus ensuring accuracy and minimizing the use of personal identifiers. Health professionals must make reasonable efforts to ensure patients understand that their data may be used in research unless they exercise their right to object. Identifiable information should not be used for research purposes if the individual has

---

[5]Medical Research Council, *Personal Information in Medical Research* (Guidelines), 1999, (s.2.2.5).

[6]British Medical Association, *Confidentiality and Disclosure of Health Information*, Oct. 14, 1999:

Confidentiality: The principle of keeping secure and secret from others, information given by or about an individual in the course of a professional relationship.

Disclosure: The revealing of identifiable health information to anyone other than the subject.

Personal health information: Any personal information relating to the physical or mental health of any person from which that person can be identified.

Anonymized information: Information, which does not, directly or indirectly, identify the person to whom it relates.

registered an objection. Nor should the contact details of potential participants in research be passed to researchers without consent.

Moreover, in these recent guidelines, the BMA has taken the explicit position that "it is not ethically necessary to seek consent to the use of anonymous information." It also maintained the position that in addition to the traditional duty of medical secrecy, "there is also strong public interest in maintaining confidentiality so that individuals will be encouraged to seek appropriate treatment and share information relevant to it." These recent guidelines repeated the concern already addressed in the 1997 Caldicott Report over the management and security of flows of information through new communication technologies. In short, the BMA maintains that the Data Protection Act of 1998 cannot adequately protect medical information.

Recently, the Medical Research Council Key Principle B maintained:

> When consent is impracticable, confidential information can be disclosed for medical research without consent if it is justified by the importance of the study; if there is no intention to contact individuals (except to seek consent) or reveal findings to them, if there are no practicable alternatives of equal effectiveness; and if the infringement of confidentiality is kept to a minimum[7]

With regard to this principle, the document notes that the "decision about whether a study is sufficiently important is not for the investigator alone, but must also be referred to a Local Research Ethics Committee for independent assessment." The techniques required for the use of personal health information in research are encoding or anonymization "so far as is reasonably possible." Anonymized data is understood as the equivalent of unidentifiable data, that are, all information that could directly identify individuals has been irreversibly removed.

A recent case of the Court of Appeal (December 21,1999)[8] reversed a High Court ruling[9] that the collection and sale of data on doctors' prescribing habits breached confidentiality even when the data are anonymized. The case hinged on the issue of implied consent to the use of anonymized data "not only by commercial companies but for public interest purposes, including medical research and statistics."[10]

The Court of Appeal held that for breach of confidence to occur the information must have: "the necessary quality of confidence about it; be imparted in circumstances imparting an obligation of confidence; and, be an unauthorized used of that information to the detriment of the party communicating it." The Court of Appeal held that due to anonymization "[t]he patient's privacy will have been safeguarded, not invaded. The pharmacist's duty of confidence will

---

[7]*Supra*, note 5.

[8]Source Informatics Limited, http://wood.ccta.gov.uk/courtser/judgeme.

[9]*R and the Department of Health (ex parte)* v. *Source Informatics* [1999] All E R 185.

[10]Dyer, C., "BMA's Patient Confidentiality Rules are Deemed Unlawful" (1999) 319 BMJ 1221.

not have been breached." It is interesting to note that albeit *in obiter,* the Court of Appeal suggested that such anonymized data would also not run afoul of articles 2(b) and 8 of the European Directive of 1995.

Australia

"The law relating to privacy in Australia is unsatisfactory. There is no general common law or statutory right to privacy. Such general privacy laws as exist have developed in a piecemeal fashion."[11]

In Australia, as in the United Kingdom, medical practitioners have no professional privilege.[12] Furthermore, any breach of confidence by a general practitioner may lead to disciplinary offenses or to civil actions rising out of tort, contract, or equity. There are also statutory provisions and guidelines imposing the requirements of confidentiality, including circumstances that constitute exceptions to confidentiality. An interesting position is that medical records are the property of the private medical practitioner who can allow or deny access (except for the Australian Capitol Territory).[13] The same does not hold for public health facilities.

The Commonwealth Privacy Act 1988 applies to research on personal information held by a Commonwealth agency. It establishes the fundamental principle related to data protection, including special provisions related to the use of identifiable personal information in medical research.[14] The Guidelines for the Protection of Privacy in the Conduct of Medical Research of the National Health and Medical Research Council (1998) not only require that each research project be approved by an institutional ethics committee but also require the following:

2.3 The written protocol for the conduct of each medical research project should state:

(d) the reasons why personal rather than de-identified information is needed;

(e) why consent to the use of personal information cannot be obtained from the individuals involved;

(j) the safeguards that will be applied to protect personal information that will be made available to other researchers or third parties.

---

[11]Chalmers, D., "Australia," in Nys Herman, (ed.) *International Encyclopedia of Laws: Medical Law,* Vol. 1 (Boston: Kluwer Law International, 1998) 1 at p. 79.

[12]*Ibid.* at p. 77: " in Victoria, Tasmania and the Northern Territory there is a privilege contained in the relevant state legislation which allows a doctor to refuse to divulge confidential information in Court proceedings unless the patient consents to the disclosure."

[13]*Breen* v. *Williams* (1996) 70 ALJR 772.

[14]Excludes states and local government, as well as private agencies.

Furthermore, the institutional ethics committee must weigh the public interest in medical research against the public interest in privacy (art. 3.2). If public interest in research substantially outweighs its interest in privacy, then the research will not be considered a breach of the Privacy Act.

France

Article 9 of the French Civil Code proclaims the right to privacy. Protection of health information, however, stems chiefly from the Penal Code (art. 226-13 and 14). This means that the sanction for breach is a criminal one, the information transmitted by the patient being of a highly personal nature (*intuitu personae*). Furthermore, whereas most obligations of a physician are what are known as "an obligation of means", medical secrecy is one of result. This is important since the ambit of the medical secret extends beyond what is heard, observed, or confided to what is understood. Thus, simple proof of breach is sufficient to constitute a fault.[15] According to the 1978 Law on Informatics, Records and Freedoms every person has the right to object to the collection and storage of personal data and to access to such data.

In a major statutory amendment in 1994 to the French omnibus data protection law,[16] French legislators set out restrictions on the automatic treatment of personal information for the purpose of health care research. This statute sets up a new body of data protection oversight, establishes substantive principles for data protection in medical research, and specifies important individual interests that must be respected before personal information can be used in a health care research project." Each request to process information for medical research is to be submitted first to the Consultative Committee on the Treatment of Information in Research Health Care sector of experts, who are then to notify the National Commission on Information and Liberties (CNIL).[17]

In 1995, the revised Code of Ethics for physicians increased the number of articles treating medical secrecy with reference to the additional conditions established by law for the protection of personal information. Disciplinary sanctions are independent of any civil or penal ones. Finally, specific laws govern not only the computerization of medical data, but also the gradual introduction of the smart card in the healthcare system.

In addition to setting up a new body of oversight, the 1994 amendment establishes important individual interests. Most important is a general requirement that personal medical information that permits the identification of individuals be encoded before transmission to a research project. Although there are excep-

---

[15]See generally, Gérard M., in *International Encyclopedia of Laws*: Medical Law, "France," *supra*, note 11, pp. 1–160, at 138–146.

[16]Computerized Processing of Name-Linked Data for the Purpose of Research in the Health Sector. Law No. 94-548.

[17]Schwartz P. M., "European Data Protection Law and Medical Privacy" at pp. 403–404 in *Genetic Secrets*, Rothstein, M., (ed.), *supra*, note 2, 1997.

tions, the law forbids the reporting of research results that permit the direct or indirect identification of concerned parties. The law also grants individuals a right to object to use of their data in any medical research project. Finally, treatment of one's health care information in a research project generally requires the individual to be personally informed of the nature of the transmitted data and his or her right to access and correct the information the intended recipient of the information and the end use (finalité) of the information.[18]

In France, the Consultative Committee on the Treatment of Information in Research and Health Care is empowered by CNIL to receive requests from researchers to use nominative information without consent, firstly, if notification of the change of recipient of nominative information would be impracticable; second, if the information is unknown to the person, and third, where the information concerns a required notifiable condition. The only restriction is that the data be coded.[19]

In 1997, the CNIL adopted Recommendation 97-008 on the treatment of personal health data. This recommendation reiterates the obligation to maintain confidentiality, and to inform the person of any transmission of information with the possibility of objection and, finally, requires the anonymization of data for any secondary uses. Where information systems involve ongoing follow-up and updating, coding, encryption, or scrambling of the information is recommended. In addition, adopting heightened security measures for medical data, the CNIL can at any time verify the respect of these conditions. Yet, the commission affirmed that in conformity with article 5 of the 1981 Convention on the Automatic Processing of Data access to nominative medical data for proper follow-up and the inclusion of such data for purposes of state social security programs, for prevention strategies, or for statistics or research were not precluded provided there is coding or anonymization.

Canada

Most Canadian jurisdictions have some form of privacy legislation in place, either as part of freedom-of-information and protection-of-privacy legislation or as a separate statute. However, in response to international developments (e.g., the 1995 European Directive) and to increasing public awareness and concern, there have been recent developments in two main areas: the expansion of legislative protection of personal information to include the private sector and the development of comprehensive legislation specific to health information. The federal Bill C-6 (formerly C-54)[20] is an example of the first; new health information legislation in Manitoba, Saskatchewan, and Alberta, and draft legislation in Ontario, are examples of the second.

---

[18]Schwartz, *ibid.* at p. 404.

[19]Art. 40-3, al. 2 of D. no. 95-682, 9 mai 1995, JO 11 mai.

[20]Bill C-6, Personal Information Protection and Electronic Documents Act, 2nd Sess., 36th Parl., 1999, Part 1.

The success of the Canada Health Infoway and similar projects under way at the national and provincial levels will depend on the development of a comprehensive and consistent legislative framework for the protection of personal health information. The Final Report of the Advisory Council on Health Infrastructure noted that "a real danger exists that Canada could end up with many different approaches to privacy and the protection of personal health information" and recommended that harmonization of provincial and federal approaches be encouraged and that "all governments in Canada should ensure that they have legislation to address privacy protection specifically aimed at protecting personal health information through explicit and transparent mechanisms."[21] In addition, it recommended that privacy legislation applicable to health information bind the public and private sectors.[22]

The legislative renewal program within Health Protection Branch Transition is another relevant part of the current legal context. The review and proposed new legislation include delineation of roles and responsibilities, division of powers, risk management, scientific freedom, and safeguards for confidentiality and privacy.[23]

There is no discrete Common Law action for breach of privacy in Canada.[24] Privacy is protected by a network of legislation, constitutional provisions, and various aspects of Common Law. Health care providers have an obligation to maintain the confidentiality of patient information as part of their duties of care and fiduciary duties.[25] A breach of privacy may also be grounds for other types of tort actions such as nuisance, trespass, libel, slander, defamation, assault, or battery.[26] If there is a contractual relationship between the provider and the patient, a duty of confidence may be considered to be implied in the contract.

In a recent case involving counselling records, the Supreme Court of Canada confirmed that section 8 of the Canadian Charter of Rights and Freedoms provides protection for such confidential information and indirectly for the therapeutic relationship.[27] In another case under the Charter, where a body sample taken without consent or for medical purposes was used in criminal pro-

---

[21]Advisory Council on Health Infrastructure, *Canada Health Infoway: Paths to Better Health*, Final Report (Health Canada Reports, February 1999), Chapter 1 at 5.2, 5.3.

[22]*Ibid.* at 5-3.

[23]Health Canada, *Shared Responsibilities, Shared Vision: Renewing the Federal Health Protection Legislation* (Discussion Paper) (Ottawa: Health Canada, 1998) at 35–36; Health Canada, *National Consultations Summary Report: Renewal of the Federal Health Protection Legislation* (Ottawa: Health Canada, 1999).

[24]For a review of Canadian law relating to health information and privacy, see Marshall M. and B. Von Tigerstrom, "Confidentiality and Disclosure of Health Information" in Downie J. and Caulfield T. (eds.), *Canadian Health Law and Policy* (Toronto: Butterworths, 1999) 143.

[25]*McInerney* v. *MacDonald*, [1992] 2 S.C.R. 138.

[26]Fridman, G.H.L., *The Law of Torts in Canada*, vol. 2 (Toronto: Carswell, 1990) at 192ff; Klar, L.N., *Tort Law*, 2d ed. (Toronto: Carswell, 1996) at 66–67.

[27]*R.* v. *Mills* [1999] S.C.J. No. 68 (QL) at para. 79–82.

ceedings, the Court held that the individual had a reasonable expectation of privacy in part because of the relationship of confidence with the health care provider.[28]

Quebec

Although not a legally recognized "state," the province of Quebec was chosen as an example of a comprehensive multilayered approach to the confidentiality of medical data within Canada. Examining the normative instruments according to their legal hierarchy, we have seen that the Canadian Charter of Rights and Freedoms contains no explicit right to privacy but has been interpreted as both a liberty interest (art. 7) and a right to be free from "unreasonable search and seizure" (art. 8).

In addition to the Canadian Charter, which serves as the ultimate filter of the constitutionality of all provincial and federal legislation, Quebec has its own charter. This Charter of Human Rights and Freedoms, which is of a quasi-constitutional nature, contains a right to respect for private life (art. 5) and more importantly the "right to nondisclosure of confidential information" even in a court of law, absent patient or statutory authorization (art. 9).

These provisions are buttressed by the Civil Code of Quebec, which since 1994 had a whole chapter with explicit provisions on the right to privacy as a right of personality. Both the Charter and the Civil Code cover governmental as well as private action.

The protection of personal information as well as access by the person is further enshrined not only in two statutes covering personal data in both the public and the private sectors[29] but also by the Act Respecting Health Services and Social Services.[30] The latter further buttresses the confidentiality of health information by requiring an explicit consent from the patient for access (art. 19). In addition, the Code of Ethics of Physicians governs the physician whether in hospital or private office and is a regulation pursuant to the act with force of law. Finally, a 1992 decision of the Supreme Court of Canada maintained that the right to information in the medical record was a personal right of the patient, although the file remained the property of the hospital.[31]

Medical files in the office of the private physician are subject to the Professions Code,[32] which requires all professional corporations to adopt a code of ethics. As mentioned, the Code of Ethics of Physicians was adopted as a regula-

---

[28]*R. v. Dyment,* [1988] 2 S.C.R. 417; *R. v. Dersch,* [1993] 3 S.C.R. 768.

[29]Act Respecting Access to Documents Held by Public Bodies and the Protection of personal information, R.S.Q., c A. 2.1; Act respecting the Protection of Personal Information in the Private Sector, R.S.Q., cp. 39.1.

[30]Act Respecting Health Services and Social Services, R.S.Q., c. S. 4.2.

[31]*McInervey* v. *MacDonald* [1992] 2 R.S.Q. 138.

[32]*Professions Code,* R.S.Q. c. C.-26.

tion pursuant to law (art. 3.01) together with the Medical Act.[33] These reinforce article 9 of the Quebec Charter concerning the quasi-constitutional duty of professional secrecy. Finally, article 35 of the Civil Code of Quebec, adopted in 1994, enunciates the right to privacy of the person and also provides recourse to an aggrieved patient in the case of treatment outside the public hospital.

As concerns research, consent (including record searches) must be free, informed, and given in writing.[34] Such consent is valid only for the period of time approved by the ethics committee (art. 19.1). An exception to this would be situations in which the director of professional services authorizes access without patient consent, according to the legislation governing access to documents held by public bodies. The researcher would have to demonstrate that the following:[35]

> 1. the intended use is not frivolous and the ends contemplated cannot be achieved otherwise, and
> 2. such nominative information will be used in a manner that ensures confidentiality.

These additional conditions of ethics approval and a determined period of time for access for research were adopted into law in January 2000 following a recent case in which access to the medical records was provided and several years later the researcher wished to continue working with patient records. Due to the merger of two hospitals, the records had been moved and the new director of professional services considered that the consent was no longer valid. The Court of Appeal however maintained that medical confidentiality was "relative" and existed primarily to benefit the patient. Since one of the aims of the research in question was to find the cause of susceptibility to manic depression and schizophrenia, the researcher needed access to the records for the purposes of familial recruitment.[35]

Iceland

On December 17, 1998, the Icelandic Parliament adopted an Act on a Health Sector Database, (Act 139/1998).[36] This act foresees the creation and operation of a centralized database containing nonpersonally identifiable clinical data. Companies can apply for a license to have access.

Article 7 of the act states that with the consent of health institutions or self-employed health care workers, data derived from medical records may be deliv-

---

[33] *Medical Act* R.S.Q. c. M.-9, art. 42.

[34] *Civil Code*, arts. 23, 24; *Act to Amend the Act Respecting Health Services and Social Services as Regards Access to Uses of Records*, art. 19.1, adopted, January 2000.

[35] *Parent* c. *Maziade* [1998] RJQ 1444–1457.

[36] *Act on a Health Sector Database, Act 139/1998*, Iceland, 1998–1999, http://brunnur.stjr.is/interpro/htr/htr.nsf/pages/gagngr-log-ensk

ered to the holder of the operating License (the "Licensee") for transfer into the Health Sector Database. The same article provides that the process shall be subject to conditions regarded as necessary by the Data Protection Commission at any time and that personal identifiers shall be encrypted before transfer to the database so that employees of the licensee work only with nonpersonally identifiable data. Personal identifiers shall be encrypted by one-way encryption, which cannot be traced back by using a cipher. The Data Protection Commission shall carry out further encryption of personal identifiers using the methods that the commission deems to ensure confidentiality best.

It is important here to underline the fact that it is employees of the health institutions in question or self-employed health workers who prepare the data for transfer to the database and not employees of the licensee.

Article 10 of the act states that the licensee is permitted to process the clinical data in the Health Sector Database derived from medical records, provided the data are processed and connected in such a way that they cannot be linked to identifiable individuals. The article provides, furthermore, that the licensee shall develop methods and protocols that meet the requirements of the Data Protection Commission in order to ensure confidentiality in connecting data from the Health Sector Database with data from a genealogical database and a genetic database.

The article furthermore provides that the licensee is not permitted to provide information on individuals and that this should be ensured (e.g., by limitation of access).

The act contains detailed provisions on monitoring, which is entrusted to three parties: (1) the Operating Committee, which shall monitor the creation and operation of the database; (2) the Data Protection Commission, which is subject to the Ministry of Justice and responsible for general surveillance of personal privacy in Iceland; and (3) an Interdisciplinary Ethics Committee, which monitors queries and research conducted using data from the Health Sector Database.

Finally, it is interesting to note that according to article 1.8, all data entering the Health Sector Database are the common property of the Icelandic nation and in the care and under the responsibility of the Minister for Health and Social Security, acting for the Icelandic government. This applies both during the time that the operating license is in effect and after its expiration.

It has been argued that this law is (not) in conformity not only with domestic law (A Special Act on the Rights of Patients, [Act 74/1997; Reg. No. 227/1991 on Medical Records and Compilation of Reports in Health Matters] pursuant to the Act on Physicians and the Act on Health Service) but also with European standards of data protection and with scientific freedom generally.[37]

On January 22 the Ministry of Health and Social Security prepared the issue of an Operating License for the Creation and Operation of a Health Sector Data-

---

[37]Arnardóttir, O.M. et al., "The Icelandic Health Sector Database" (1999) *6 European Journal Health Law*, 307–362. For a critique of the database, see Roscam Abbing, H., "Central Health Database in Iceland and Patient's Rights," (1999) 6 *European Journal of Health Law*, 363–371.

base of nonidentifiable health information. The licensee is authorized to convert information in the Health Sector Database with a genetic database with the approval of the Data Protection Commission.

No genetic information or samples can be obtained for research purposes without specific patient consent. It goes without saying, however, that any such information found in the medical record would automatically be in the Health Sector Database unless the patient has exercised the opting-out provision.

CONCLUSION

Given the often eclectic if not confusing state of the law due to the combined effect of privacy, medical confidentiality, and personal data protection, it is difficult to draw any conclusions except perhaps to argue for the consolidation and harmonization of health data protection. This situation occurs because although the trends in all three sectors are welcome, their combined effect creates uncertainty since it is not always clear which rules apply. Moreover, most countries also provide for recourse to overarching constitutional protection, or in the absence of such, to human rights legislation be it national or regional as in Europe. Such consolidation and clarification including the ambit of legitimate exceptions would not only be welcome but perhaps serve as a first step towards an international "charter" on health information.

Furthermore, we are now witnessing a further expansion of health information protection and promotion in the emergence of the right not to know and in the area of research in the move from coding or encryption to anonymization. Both of these recent developments are not without implications, the individual having been effectively removed from ongoing communication of health information. Four questions remain: (1) What degree of informed consent is required for the valid exercise of the "right not to know." (2) Will anonymization although legally and ethically expedient, ultimately harm good science? (3) In the long run, will both impede identification for follow-up for proper medical treatment? (4) If so, have we unwittingly created a system of overprotection of the individual to the detriment of population health through prevention?

Moreover, in this search for guidance and clarity, health information should be distinguished from the sometimes-draconian overreach of personal data protection often aimed at thwarting access by commercial bodies. The indiscriminate application of this legislation when combined with the moral or legal force of medical codes of ethics can indirectly harm individual health to say nothing of blocking the state's legitimate role in health systems planning. The majority of countries studied here cannot properly fulfill this latter obligation. In the rush to promote individual privacy and autonomy with regard to health information, we may have lost sight of the larger picture of the health of society and that of future generations.

Biographical Sketches

BERNARD LO (*Chair*), is professor of medicine and director of the Program in Medical Ethics at the University of California, San Francisco. He chairs the End of Life Committee convened by the American College of Physicians - American Society of Internal Medicine, which is developing consensus recommendations for clinical care near the end of life. He directs the national coordinating office for the Initiative to Strengthen the Patient - Provider Relationship in a Changing Health Care Environment, funded by the Robert Wood Johnson Foundation. He also directs the Ethics Core of the Center for AIDS Prevention Studies at UCSF. Dr. Lo is a member of the National Bioethics Advisory commission and of the Data Safety Monitoring Board for the AIDS Clinical Trials Group at the National Institute of Allergy and Infectious Diseases. He is a member of the Institute of Medicine and chairs the IOM Board on Health Sciences Policy. Dr. Lo has written more than 100 articles in peer-reviewed medical journals, on such issues as decisions about life-sustaining interventions, decision-making for incompetent patients, physician-assisted suicide, and ethical issues regarding HIV infection. He is the author of *Resolving Ethical Dilemmas: A Guide for Clinicians*, a comprehensive analysis of ethical dilemmas in adult medicine. He is also a practicing general internist who teaches clinical medicine to residents and medical students.

ELIZABETH B. ANDREWS, M.P.H., Ph.D., directs the Worldwide Epidemiology Department at Glaxo Wellcome, based in Research Triangle Park, North Carolina and Greenford, England. The epidemiology program encompasses epidemiologic research on safety, natural history of disease, disease burden, and general descriptive epidemiology. She is currently president of the International Society for Pharmacoepidemiology, an organization broadly representative of government, industry, and academic researchers. Dr. Andrews serves as adjunct associate professor of epidemiology at the University of North Carolina (UNC) School of Public Health. She participates as a member of the Pharmaceutical Research and Manufacturers of America Clinical Safety Surveillance Committee and for three years chaired its Epidemiology Subcommittee. She is a member of the editorial board of the journal *Pharmacoepidemiology and Drug Safety*. She serves on the governing board of the UNC School of Public Health's Public Health Foundation. In addition, she serves on the Advisory Panel on Research of the Association of American Medical Colleges and the Data Privacy Working Group of the European Federation of Pharmaceutical Industries and Associations. She also serves on the Food and Drug Administration's Reproductive Health Drugs Advisory Committee's Subcommittee on Pregnancy Labeling. Over the past two years, she has testified on medical records confidentiality before the U.S. Senate and House committees and the National Committee on Vital and Health Statistics. Dr. Andrews received her master's in public health and health policy and administration and Ph.D. in epidemiology from the University of North Carolina School of Public Health. Prior to joining Burroughs Wellcome in 1982, she managed the Statewide Regionalized Perinatal Care Program and directed the Purchase-of-Care Services for the State Health Department of North Carolina.

JOHN COLMERS is executive director of the Maryland Health Care Commission (MHCC), an agency created through the merger of two existing health regulatory commissions. MHCC is charged with health care reform activities for the state, the development and adoption of a state health plan, and the compilation and analysis of health care datasets, among other responsibilities. Prior to the merger, Mr. Colmers was executive director of the Health Care Access and Cost Commission (HCACC), one of the organizations in the merger. The HCACC implemented many initiatives, including report cards providing information on the quality and performance of health maintenance organizations and standards for the operation of electronic health networks. Before this, Mr. Colmers was the executive director of the Health Services Cost Review Commission, overseeing Maryland's all-payer hospital rate setting system. Mr. Colmers did undergraduate work at Johns Hopkins University, received his master of public health from the University of North Carolina, and has returned to Johns Hopkins University for doctoral study of health services research.

GEORGE T. DUNCAN is professor of statistics in the H. John Heinz III School of Public Policy and Management and the Department of Statistics at Carnegie Mellon University. His current research work centers on information technology and social accountability, especially on confidentiality issues. He chaired the Panel on Confidentiality and Data Access of the Commission on Behavioural and Social Sciences and Education (CBSSE) Committee on National Statistics, which resulted in the report, *Private Lives and Public Policies: Confidentiality and Accessibility of Government Statistics.* He chaired the American Statistical Association's Committee on Privacy and Confidentiality. He served on the American Medical Association's Expert Advisory Panel on Privacy and Confidentiality. He has been editor of the Theory and Methods Section of the *Journal of the American Statistical Association.* He is a fellow of the American Statistical Association, an elected member of the International Statistical Institute, and a fellow of the American Association for the Advancement of Science.

JANLORI GOLDMAN directs the Health Privacy Project at Georgetown University's Institute for Health Care Research and Policy. The project is dedicated to ensuring that people's privacy is safeguarded in the health care environment. In 1997, Ms. Goldman was a visiting scholar at Georgetown University Law Center. In 1994, Ms. Goldman cofounded the Center for Democracy and Technology, a nonprofit civil liberties organization committed to preserving free speech and privacy on the Internet. Ms. Goldman also worked at the Electronic Frontier Foundation in 1994. From 1986 to 1994, Ms. Goldman was the staff attorney and director of the Privacy and Technology Project of the American Civil Liberties Union (ACLU). While at the ACLU, Ms. Goldman led the effort to enact the Video Privacy Protection Act and led efforts to protect people's health, credit and financial information, and personal information held by the government. She was the legislative director of the Minnesota affiliate of the ACLU from 1984 to 1986. Ms. Goldman has testified frequently before the U.S. Congress and served on numerous commissions and advisory boards. Her publications include "A Federal Right of Information Privacy," coauthored with Jerry Berman and included as a chapter in *Computers, Ethics, and Social Values* (ed. Helen Nissenbaum, Prentice Hall, 1995); *Privacy and Health Information Systems: A Guide to Protecting Patient Confidentiality,* coauthored with Deirdre Mulligan (Foundation for Health Care Quality, 1996); "Protecting Privacy to Improve Health Care," which appeared in *Health Affairs,* (November - December1998); and *Promoting Health/Protecting Privacy: A Primer,* coauthored with Zoe Hudson for the California Health Care Foundation and Consumers Union. The Health Privacy Project also recently released two reports: *The State of Health Privacy: An Uneven Terrain/A Comprehensive Survey of State Health Privacy Statutes and Best Principles for Health Privacy: A Report of the Health Privacy Working Group.*

CRAIG WALTER HENDRIX is associate professor of medicine, Division of Clinical Pharmacology, Department of Medicine, Johns Hopkins University School of Medicine, where he is currently director of the Johns Hopkins' University Drug Development Unit. He also holds joint appointments in pharmacology and molecular sciences and epidemiology. He earned his M.D. at Georgetown University School of Medicine followed by postdoctoral training at Johns Hopkins Hospital. He is board-certified in internal medicine and infectious diseases. His clinical research has focused on HIV epidemiology and prevention within military populations and clinical pharmacology of antiretroviral drugs. Dr. Hendrix is invited to lecture worldwide on HIV impact, prevention and treatment. His university service includes membership on the Johns Hopkins University School of Medicine institutional review board.

MARK C. HORNBROOK, a health economist by training, is an associate director and senior investigator at the Kaiser Permanente Center for Health Research (CHR). He leads the center's program in economic, social, and health services research and is a member of the senior management team at CHR. His current research focuses on payment systems for HMOs under private and public health insurance programs. With support from the Health Care Financing Administration, the Robert Wood Johnson Foundation, and Kaiser Permanente, he is developing morbidity-based risk assessment models to adjust payments to health plans to counter selection bias. He is also developing and simulating a new risk contracting payment system for Medicare based on competitive market premiums rather than Medicare fee-for-service payments. Previously, with support from Kaiser Foundation Health Plan, Dr. Hornbrook developed health care expense forecasting models using the SF-36 and the Medicare Current Beneficiary Survey. Dr. Hornbrook directs the CHR Economics Core in conducting a series of economic evaluations of several innovative disease management, disease prevention, and health care delivery programs related to long-term care of frail elderly, smoking cessation, cancer screening, mental illness, and childhood asthma, and other studies as well. Dr. Hornbrook received a master's degree in economics from the University of Denver in 1969 and a Ph.D. in medical care organization, with emphasis in health economics, from the University of Michigan in 1975. Currently, Dr. Hornbrook chairs the Scientific Review and Evaluation Board of the Health Services Research and Development Service, Department of Veterans Affairs. He also is a member of the Measures Council of the Foundation for Accountability. He was named a fellow in the Association for Health Services Research in 1996.

LISA I. IEZZONI is professor of medicine at Harvard Medical School and co-director of research in the Division of General Medicine and Primary Care, Department of Medicine, at Beth Israel Deaconess Medical Center in Boston. She received her degrees in medicine and health policy and management from Harvard University. Dr. Iezzoni has conducted numerous studies for the Agency for Health Care Policy and Research, the Health Care Financing Administration, and private foundations on a variety of topics, including the use of clinical data to predict hospitalization costs and patient outcomes, comparing severity of illness across teaching and nonteaching hospitals, evaluating the utility of severity information for quality assessment, identifying complications of care using administrative data, and using information from hospital data systems to predict patient clinical and functional outcomes. She has published and spoken widely on measurement of the severity of illness and has edited a textbook on risk adjustment for measuring health care outcomes. A 1996 recipient of the investigator Award in Health Policy Research sponsored by Robert Wood Johnson Foundation, she is studying disability policy issues relating to mobility impairments. Dr. Iezzoni is on the editorial boards of major medical health services research journals, and she serves on the National Committee on Vital and Health Statistics and the Board of Directors of the National Forum for Health Care Quality Measurement and Reporting.

DONALD KORNFELD is associate dean of the Faculty of Medicine of the Columbia University College of Medicine, and professor of psychiatry and attending psychiatrist at Columbia Presbyterian Hospital. He served for six years as chairman of the Institutional Review Board at the N.Y. State Psychiatric Institute and since 1991 has been Chairman of the Columbia Presbyterian Medical Center Institutional Review Board. He is director of the Consultation/Liaison and Behavioral Medicine Service at the Columbia Presbyterian Medical Center and was a member of the first ethics committee established there. He has published on a wide variety of psychiatric problems and ethical issues related to medicine and surgery. He is a fellow of the American Psychiatric Association and a past president of the American Psychosomatic Society.

ELLIOT STONE has been executive director and Corporate Eexecutive Officer of the Massachusetts Health Data Consortium since it was established in 1978 as a private, nonprofit corporation. The consortium is a neutral setting for the collection and analysis of large health care databases. The consortium publishes annual reports on hospital prices, utilization, and communities' hospital dependency to a broad constituency of health care organizations and business coalitions, and provides data and technical support to health services researchers. In 1994, Mr. Stone organized the Affiliated Health Information Networks of New England project to improve the state's electronic health care information infrastructure among health plans and providers through standards required by the federal Health Insurance Portability and Accountability. Mr. Stone served on the Institute of Medicine's Committee on Regional Health Data Networks, which published *Health Data in the Information Age: Use, Disclosure and Privacy*. He was a member of the Committee to Study National Cryptography Policy for the National Research Council and the National Academy of Science's Computer Science and Telecommunications Board and provided financial support for the NRC study *For the Record: Protecting Electronic Health Information*.

PETER SZOLOVITS is professor of computer science and engineering in the Michigan Instutute of Technology (MIT) Department of Electrical Engineering and Computer Science and director of the Clinical Decision-Making Group within the MIT Laboratory for Computer Science. His research centers on the application of artificial intelligence (AI) methods to problems of medical decision making and design of information systems for health care institutions and patients. He has worked on problems of diagnosis, therapy planning, execution, and monitoring for various medical conditions; computational aspects of genetic counseling; controlled sharing of health information; and privacy and confidentiality issues in medical record systems. His interests in AI include knowledge representation, qualitative reasoning, and probabilistic inference. His interests in medical computing include Web-based heterogeneous medical record systems, lifelong personal health information systems, and design of cryptographic schemes for health identifiers. He teaches classes in artificial intelligence, programming languages, medical computing, medical decision making, knowledge-based systems, and probabilistic inference. Professor Szolovits has been on the editorial board of several journals, has served as program chairman and on the program committees of national conferences, and has been a founder of and consultant for several companies that apply AI to problems of commercial interest, including W3Health, which develops Web-based solutions for connecting the health care community. He served on the Committee on Maintaining Privacy and Security in Health Care Applications on the National Information Infrastructure, which produced the NRC report *For the Record.*

ADELE A. WALLER, J.D., is a partner and member of the Health Law Group with the Chicago law firm of Bell, Boyd and Lloyd. A substantial portion of her practice involves advising clients on legal issues related to health information technology. Ms. Waller has spoken extensively on health information technology law issues for organizations such as the American Bar Association, the American Health Lawyers Association, American Health Information Management Association, University Health System Consortium, Association for Health Services Research, and the Healthcare Information Management Systems Society. She has published numerous articles and book chapters on health information technology law topics. Ms. Waller serves on the Board of Directors of the American Health Lawyers Association, chairs its annual Health Information and Technology Conference, and served in the leadership of its Health Information and Technology Substantive Law Committee from 1994 to 1999. She is a member of on the Editorial Advisory Board of CCH Compliance and of the Editorial Board of Aspen Publishing's *Managed Care Law Manual.* Ms. Waller is a member of the adjunct faculty of the University of Illinois at Chicago and has been an adjunct faculty member for the Health Law Institute at the Loyola University of Chicago School of Law.

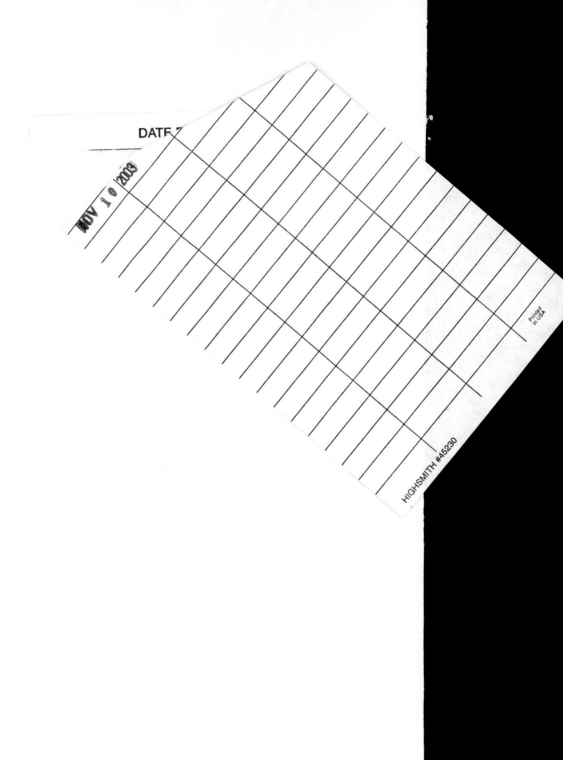

DATE